Chair Yoga and Beyond

A Comprehensive Chair-Based Fitness
Guide for Seniors

Sally Harmon

Table of Contents

Introduction

If you want something you never had, you must be willing to do something you've never done. –Thomas Jefferson

Have you ever wondered how you can maintain agility in your golden years and reverse the effects of aging to fully embrace and enjoy life? You can live a fulfilling life by prioritizing your physical and mental health. With regular exercise and a healthy diet, you can unlock the keys to vitality and longevity and pave the way to a life filled with peace, good health, and happiness. After all, the ultimate aspiration of every individual is to discover fulfillment and contentment. Achieving such satisfaction is possible when you are healthy and strong—both mentally and physically.

Yoga harmonizes your mind, body, and soul through physical postures called asanas, deep breathing exercises called pranayama, and hand gestures called mudras. It is an age-old practice that originated in ancient India. The ancient scriptures explain yogic philosophy and the exercises that serve as timeless guides for holistic well-being and spiritual growth. Over the years, yoga practitioners have innovated and adapted yoga exercises to foster inclusivity and accessibility to ensure its benefits reach individuals of all abilities. Chair yoga is one such example. It makes yoga accessible to people who face mobility and balance issues and those who have suffered from an injury or experience pain that has led to a less active lifestyle, including seniors. In such cases, sitting on a chair while exercising can be much more comfortable than sitting on a yoga mat or standing.

Chair yoga can effectively help you control your health and well-being if you set realistic goals, exercise regularly, keep track of your progress, and challenge yourself a bit more every day. So let's start a stimulating journey into chair-based fitness by exploring the numerous benefits of seated exercise.

Many yogis have tried to redefine yoga to encompass not just physical postures but also mindfulness, breath work, and ethical principles, aiming for a more holistic approach to well-being and self-discovery. Here is a brief description of the different yoga styles (McGee, 2022):

- **Hatha yoga:** Focuses on physical postures and breathing exercises to promote balance and relaxation.

- **Restorative yoga:** Focuses on relaxation and healing through gentle poses supported by props to help you get deep rest and feel rejuvenated.

- **Vinyasa yoga:** Emphasizes flowing sequences of poses synchronized with breath to promote fluidity of movement.

- **Kundalini yoga:** Incorporates dynamic movements, breathing techniques, and meditation to awaken energy within the body.

- **Yin yoga:** Involves holding passive poses for extended periods to target deep connective tissues and improve flexibility.

- **Iyengar yoga:** Involves holding poses for longer durations with precise alignment and the use of props like blocks, belts, and blankets to develop strength, flexibility, and stability while also refining body awareness and concentration.

Depending on your fitness goals, you can follow a specific yoga style or integrate different styles to derive a wide range of benefits. Some yoga styles may not be suitable for seniors, such as Ashtanga yoga and power yoga, which involve dynamic poses, and hot yoga, which consists of a series of 26 poses practiced in a heated room to enhance detoxification and flexibility. Consult with a healthcare professional and a qualified yoga instructor to determine which type of yoga is safe for your needs and abilities.

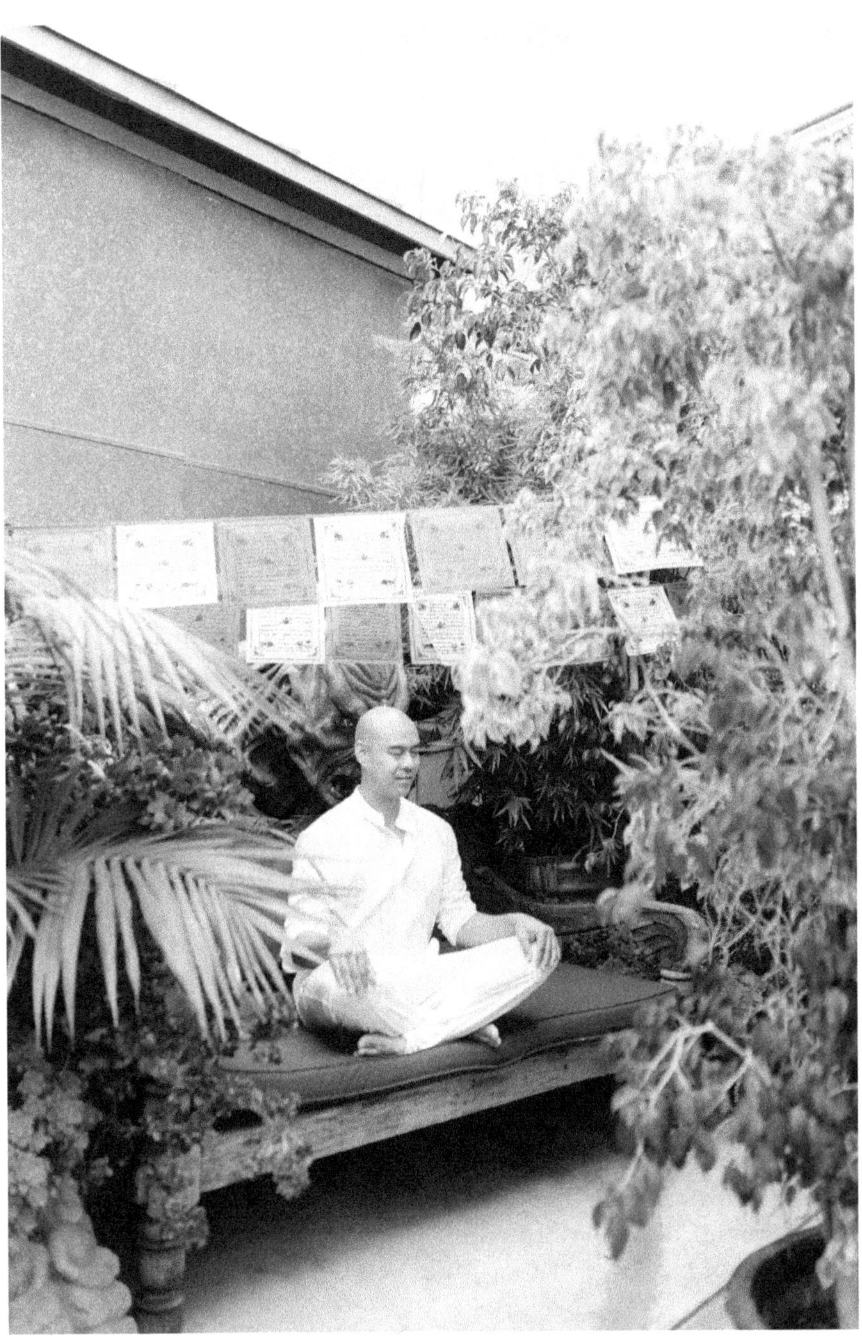

Chair Yoga: Definition, Origin, and Principles

Yoga is for everyone, and there is no better way to make its benefits accessible for all than through chair yoga. It is not about stressing yourself to reach the perfect pose but about exercising your muscles and joints, relaxing your mind, and keeping yourself active and healthy.

Chair yoga can be defined as a modification of traditional yoga that involves the use of a chair to perform the exercises in a seated position or to use it for support while performing standing poses. This wonderful yoga technique was developed by Lakshmi Voelker, a yoga therapist, in 1982 (Kain, n.d.).

Although chair yoga is suitable for those who have recovered from an injury or find mat practice difficult because of pain or a health condition like arthritis, anyone can benefit from this practice (Helmer, n.d.). Chair yoga is low-impact and as effective as traditional yoga, and once you improve your flexibility, balance, and strength with gentle chair yoga, you can advance to the next level, which includes standing poses using the chair as a support.

Yoga also involves lying poses. You may perform such poses on your bed if not on a yoga mat. This gentle variant of yoga also suits people facing mobility issues, knee discomfort, or back pain.

Yoga offers a range of exercises that enable your muscles and joints to attain their full range of motion. As we reach the age of 60, our stamina and muscular strength reduce naturally, leading to pain, tiredness, and even reduced mobility.

Chair yoga can help improve your mobility and provides hope and tangible improvements for those who find it challenging to bend or sit on the ground. You do not need to worry about hurting your knees or stressing your back while sitting on or getting up from the ground.

Be Open and Creative and Integrate Yoga With Other Disciplines

Yoga involves a spectrum of exercises ranging from gentle to intense, so you can customize your workout according to your mobility, flexibility, and stamina to ensure your safety and wellness. As you advance in your practice, you can introduce gradual challenges to foster continuous growth and improvement. In addition, you can also combine yoga exercises with other disciplines to derive holistic benefits.

Yoga encompasses various strength-building exercises such as boat pose, cobra pose, and squats, heart-healthy exercise sequences like sun salutations and bow pose, and numerous exercises that are used by Pilates practitioners too. Practicing simple cardio and strength training exercises along with yoga can help you maximize your workouts and speed up the strengthening of your muscles and stabilizing of your core. This book offers guidance on practicing chair yoga and chair variations of cardio, strength training, and Pilates exercises to provide you with a variety of movements that can bring you holistic wellness. So even when life seems overwhelming, push yourself a bit, keep exercising, and face every obstacle with a positive outlook.

By incorporating diverse exercises into your yoga routine, you engage different muscle groups, enhance flexibility, and improve overall physical fitness. This multifaceted approach not only promotes harmony and balance within the body but also fosters mental clarity and emotional equilibrium as you center your mind to perform each exercise well. Breathing deeply also signals the brain that "all is well" and helps you stay in the present moment.

Chair-Based Fitness and Its Advantages

Chair-based exercises offer countless benefits for your mind and body. Let's take a look at a few of the things you can gain from engaging in chair-based fitness:

- **Chair exercises strengthen your muscles and joints:** Chair yoga is as good as traditional yoga for improving muscle strength, balance, posture, and gait, which helps enhance confidence and independence (*Chair Yoga*, 2023). Seated cardio and Pilates are also proven to be as effective as their traditional counterparts.

- **Chair-based fitness routines can reduce pain and stress:** Any form of exercise stimulates the release of your body's natural painkillers, endorphins. When you have knee or back pain, heart ailments, or any factor that impacts your lifestyle and causes you to be less active, you are more prone to feel weak and mentally stressed doing nothing. Performing chair yoga exercises sends signals to your brain to release endorphins, relieving body aches and discomfort. Exercise equipment as simple as a chair can help you live a more active lifestyle and give you a feeling of accomplishment, which stimulates dopamine production, and dopamine reduces stress. People of all ages and fitness levels can perform gentle chair yoga and derive its benefits (*Chair Yoga*, 2023).

- **Seated exercises help manage stiffness and arthritis symptoms:** Joint stiffness and arthritis pain can make sitting on a yoga mat or standing up from the ground challenging. Chair yoga can help you maintain your exercise routine and manage arthritis symptoms like joint pain and stiffness by stimulating blood flow and synovial fluid circulation between joints.

- **Exercising while seated helps prevent injuries:** As long as you perform chair exercises while seated on a stable, sturdy chair, there is less risk of falls and injuries.

- **Chair-based workouts improve sleep:** You may not be getting enough quality sleep due to hormonal issues, pain and stiffness in joints, or the side effects of certain medicines. These problems may be aggravated by a sedentary lifestyle. However, if you start exercising from the comfort of a chair, your health issues may improve. Even seated exercises can help enhance blood circulation, regulate hormone levels, and provide relaxation, leading to better sleep.

Exercise Safely

Start with simple exercises and increase the intensity and duration gradually while listening to your body's signals to avoid injury and promote long-term well-being. Here are a few more tips to ensure your safety while exercising:

- **Always prioritize your health, comfort, and safety while exercising:** Exercise is meant to help you enjoy better health, so it should not cause pain or discomfort. Be responsive to such signals and stop exercising if you start experiencing pain or discomfort beyond the normal exertion associated with exercise. Continuing to exercise despite such signals can lead to injuries and other health issues. It's important to listen to your body and adjust your workout accordingly to ensure a safe and enjoyable exercise experience.

- **Consult your healthcare provider:** It's important to consult your physician before beginning a new type of exercise, especially if you are on medication or are dealing with an injury or health issue. You may also consult a fitness expert or healthcare provider for personalized advice, precautions, guidance, and support even if you aren't facing any specific health issues. If you experience pain or injury as a result of exercising, it's advisable to consult a healthcare professional.

- **Keep yourself well-hydrated:** Typically, you should aim to drink at least eight to ten glasses of water a day, but it is important to note that this is a general guideline and some individuals may require more or less water intake based on their specific needs. You should also drink at least one glass of water an hour before exercising so your body does not get dehydrated during the workout. Not drinking enough water can be detrimental to physical and mental functioning.

- **Eat at least two hours before exercising:** Eat a light meal or snack at least two hours before your workout to provide you with energy without causing discomfort during physical activity. This allows for proper digestion and helps prevent issues such as indigestion or cramping, promoting a more comfortable and enjoyable workout.

- **Use a sturdy chair:** A comfortable, sturdy chair is safe for exercising and should preferably have a backrest but no arms to allow for a wider range of arm and upper body movement while exercising.

- **Use yoga aids for extra comfort:** For some yoga poses, you may keep a folded blanket or yoga mat under your feet for comfort or place a cushion at your back for support. Yoga straps aid smooth movement while stretching, and yoga blocks help with exercises that require you to touch the ground by decreasing the distance between your fingers and the ground. These tools can help you achieve poses you might not otherwise be able to.

- **Modify your exercises to meet your individual abilities and limits:** If you have knee or back problems, sitting or lying on a yoga mat may be difficult. Using a chair for seated exercises and a bed for lying poses requires you to make some modifications to ensure safety and effectiveness.

Chair Yoga and Beyond is a complete guide designed to provide accessible and inclusive fitness routines specifically for seniors or people with mobility issues to improve mobility, strength, and overall well-being. When yoga is creatively and methodically combined with cardiovascular exercises, Pilates, and strength training, they complement one another and can enhance your overall well-being more efficiently. Cardiovascular exercises improve your heart rate and blood circulation, while strength training exercises involve working against your body weight or external resistance to maintain or improve your muscle mass and bone health. Pilates, a mind-body exercise, tones your muscles, improves your kinesthetics, strengthens your core, and enhances mobility.

Keep reading to learn more about these various exercise disciplines and to gain an understanding of their transformative power to enhance your well-being and help you live a fulfilling and independent life. So what are you waiting for? Get ready to take control of your life with this everlasting and enjoyable fitness journey!

Chapter 1:

Chair Yoga Magic

You're never so old that it's OK to be weak. —Bill Curry

Have you ever wondered how a simple chair could be a source of power, independence, and good health? Whether your joints are stiff or your knees or back hurt, easy poses performed on a chair provide convenience, relaxation, and flexibility, so find a quiet spot in your home to keep a stable, comfortable, and armless chair for exercising.

Exploring the Possibilities of Chair Yoga

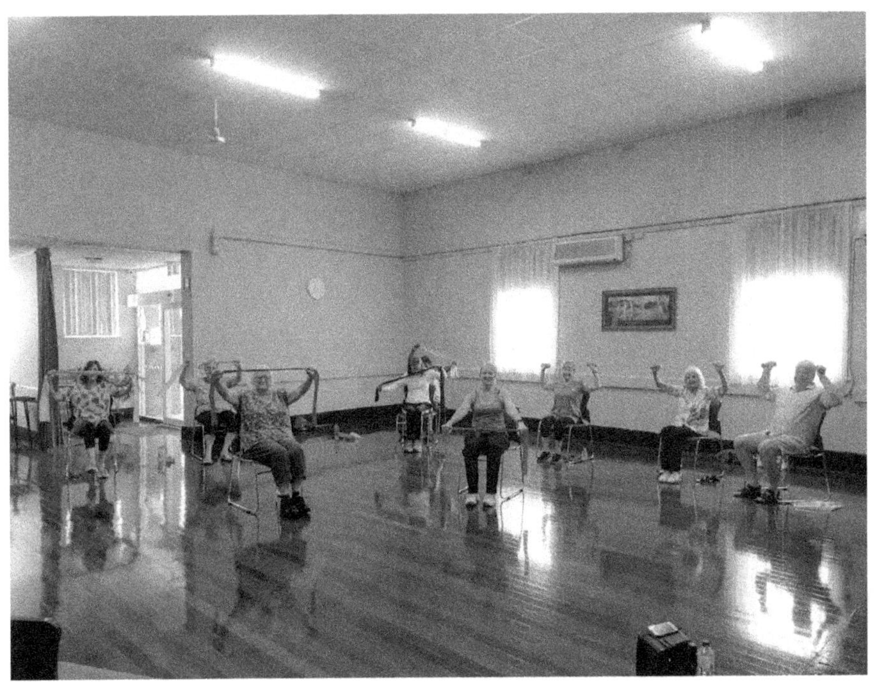

Yoga includes the asanas (physical postures), pranayama (breath control), dhyana (meditation), and relaxation techniques. Some mudras, or hand gestures, are useful while meditating. In chair yoga, you follow the same principles as in traditional yoga, like staying in the moment, focusing on your breath, and forming the correct pose. Only necessary modifications are made to the poses to adapt them to the seated position (Helmer, n.d.).

Studies show chair yoga improves seniors' mobility and functional fitness (Yao et al., 2023). Chair-based workouts can be tailored to various fitness levels, skills, and mobility limitations, making the benefits of the exercises accessible to many people. Integrating other chair exercises can also increase your strength and mobility. Let's see how we can explore chair yoga and tailor it to our needs:

- **Add variety and fun to your workout:** Other than integrating a wide range of chair-based workouts like strength training and cardio with yoga, you can play music, beautify your exercise corner by placing some plants in your space, or simply let the sunshine in by opening the curtains.

- **Be adaptable:** Gradually challenging yourself by trying new exercises is important for continued progress. For instance, when you notice an improvement in your flexibility when performing basic stretching exercises like finger stretch, arm stretch, and leg extensions consistently, you may move on to try exercises like forward fold or downward dog that involve core muscles. Once you notice more improvement over time, you can try standing poses using a wall or chair for support. After that, you can use external weights to intensify your workout, and so on.

- **Practice chair yoga regularly:** The comfort and suitability of chair workouts enable you to exercise regularly, whether at home, work, or while traveling.

- **Have a positive attitude:** Incorporating exercise into your daily routine can seem difficult at first, but once you develop a habit, you will start to see positive changes in your strength, flexibility, and balance. Embrace chair-based fitness with curiosity and an open mind and see it as a chance for growth and transformation.

- **Develop reasonable and attainable fitness goals:** To derive maximum health and fitness benefits, whether it's improving flexibility, increasing strength, or simply remaining active, you should have clear objectives in mind.

- **Use yoga props for challenging poses:** Props like cushions, bolsters, yoga straps, and yoga blocks provide support, stability, and alignment assistance, enabling practitioners to explore poses more deeply, refine alignment, and access postures that might otherwise be too challenging. By incorporating props into your yoga routine, you can intensify your workout, deepen stretches, and cultivate a broader understanding of yoga's principles.

So be positive, notice your progress, and celebrate small victories along the journey.

Chair Asanas for Beginners

In this section, we'll look at some basic chair exercises that you can perform as a beginner.

Seated Neck Stretches

1. Turn your head as far as is comfortable to one side and hold for a moment.

2. Return to center then repeat the motion on the other side.

3. Repeat the exercise 4–6 times on both sides.

Benefits:

- Neck stretches tone the muscles in the neck.

- They help relieve pain and stiffness in the neck.

Seated Neck Rotations

1. Tilt your head slowly to one side, bringing your ear toward your shoulder.

2. Slowly roll your head toward the center of your body, bringing your chin to your chest.

3. Lift your chin back up to look forward again before repeating the motion on the other side.

4. Do 3–4 of these neck rotations on each side.

Benefits:

- Neck rotations promote relaxation in the neck muscles.

- They help reduce neck pain and stiffness.

Seated Mountain Pose (Tadasana)

1. Sit in an upright position on your chair with your feet on the floor about shoulder-width apart.

2. Rest your hands on your thighs.

3. Extend your spine, reaching the top of your head toward the ceiling.

4. Be sure your shoulders are relaxed and away from your ears as you stretch your spine.

5. Close your eyes and take a few deep breaths, grounding yourself in this posture before relaxing again.

Benefits:

- Seated mountain pose helps align the spine, promoting better posture by strengthening the muscles along the back and core.

- This pose can flex your spine, shoulders, and hips.

- Holding the pose requires concentration, which can help sharpen mental focus and promote mindfulness.

- The gentle stretching and focus on breathing can help alleviate stress and promote relaxation.

- This pose engages various muscle groups, including the core, back, and shoulders, increasing strength and stability.

- The gentle compression of the abdomen in this exercise can aid digestion and relieve discomfort.

- Seated mountain pose promotes heart health.

Seated Side Stretch

1. Sit upright on your chair with your back straight.

2. Raise your right arm overhead as you inhale deeply.

3. Hold the chair's side with your left hand for support or place it on your thigh.

4. Reach your right arm and tilt your body to the left, stretching along your right side.

5. Hold the stretch for a count of 5 before returning to center.

6. Repeat on the other side, inhaling as you raise your left arm and stretch to the right.

Benefits:

- Side stretches stretch the waist, ribcage, shoulders, and neck.

- They increase flexibility in the spine.

- They help relax your shoulders and neck and improve posture.

- This exercise stimulates digestion.

- Side stretches enhance breathing capacity and promote relaxation.

- They can help alleviate stress and anxiety.

Some Basic Asanas You Can Perform on Your Bed

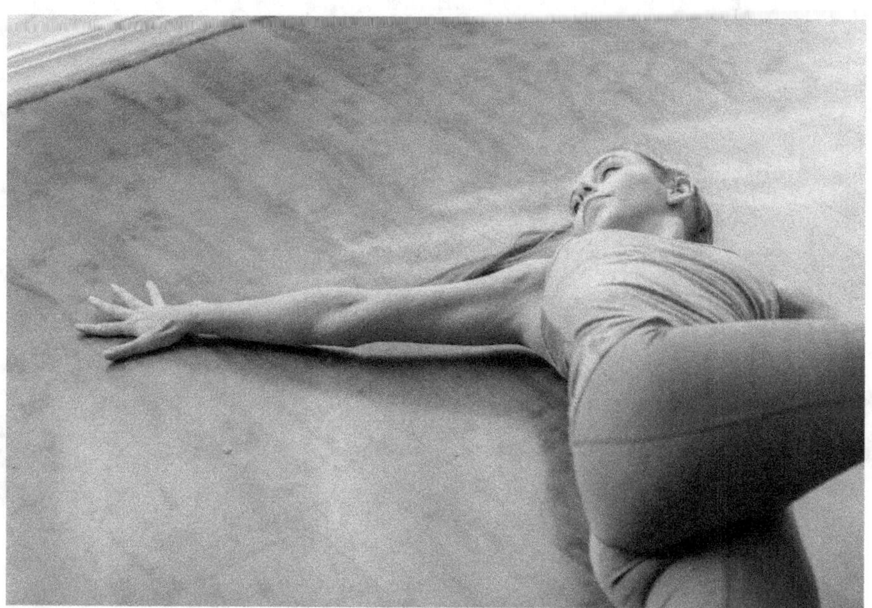

You can practice many yoga poses on a chair, but yoga includes lying poses as well, which are usually done on a yoga mat. If you find it difficult to perform them on a mat, you can perform them on your bed instead to derive their benefits.

Supine Knee-to-Chest Pose (Apanasana)

1. Lie on your back on your bed with your knees bent and feet flat on the bed.

2. Breathe deeply as you bring your right knee toward your chest. Use both hands to hold your knee and feel the stretch in your lower back and hips.

3. Keep breathing deeply as you hold the stretch for a count of 5-10.

4. Switch legs and repeat on the left side.

Benefits:

- Apanasana gently stretches the lower back muscles, releasing tension and alleviating discomfort.

- This pose can aid in digestion and relieve bloating or discomfort.

- By gently opening the hips and stretching the hip flexors, this pose can release tension accumulated from prolonged sitting or physical activity.

- Practicing Apanasana before bed can help relax the body and mind, making it easier to fall asleep and improving sleep quality.

Supine Spinal Twist

1. Lie on your back, bend your knees, and keep your feet flat on the bed.

2. Extend your arms out to the sides in a T position, palms facing down.

3. Inhale and exhale as you gently drop both knees to one side, keeping your shoulders flat on the bed.

4. Turn your head and look in the opposite direction of your knees, feeling a gentle twist in your spine.

5. Hold for a count of 10, then move your knees back to center.

6. Repeat on the other side.

Benefits:

- Supine spinal twists gently stretch and release tension in the muscles along the spine, promoting flexibility and relaxation and reducing discomfort.

- The twisting action can massage the abdominal organs, aiding digestion and promoting digestive health.

- Practicing this exercise regularly can reduce back pain.

You may have experienced those lazy mornings where you want to stay in bed even though it's getting late, but here's an interesting way to say goodbye to the morning blues: Start by being grateful to the Almighty and say a prayer. Gently twist and stretch your fingers and toes while taking deep breaths. This is how you can incorporate lying poses into your daily routine and get up in the morning feeling more energized. You will come out of sleepy mode and start feeling positive and ready to face whatever the day has in store for you. You can then get ready to do some basic chores, drink water, have a light breakfast, and perform chair exercises. With a consistent yoga practice, you will soon find fun in being flexible and independent.

Chapter 2:

The Fun of Flexibility

Rigidity invites vulnerability; flexibility breeds adaptability. –Aloo Denish Obiero

A flexible body allows your muscles and joints to reach their full range of motion, while a flexible mind allows your thoughts to evolve over time. Evolution is the way of life. The more you embrace and adapt to changes, the more you evolve into a better version of yourself as each experience becomes a life lesson. Conversely, rigidity can hinder personal growth and contribute to deteriorating health. Therefore, if you are mentally and physically flexible, you can enjoy the fun that follows.

When you exercise regularly, connections are established between your muscles and nerve cells. This phenomenon is called muscle memory. It's the reason a child who learns how to swim at a young age doesn't forget the skill as they grow up. The sequence of movements practiced numerous times is retained in the nerve cells, making it easier to recall and perform the learned skill. This means that the more regularly you exercise, the better your muscle memory becomes, leading to smoother and more efficient execution of daily tasks and activities.

Enhance Your Health With Yoga Stretches

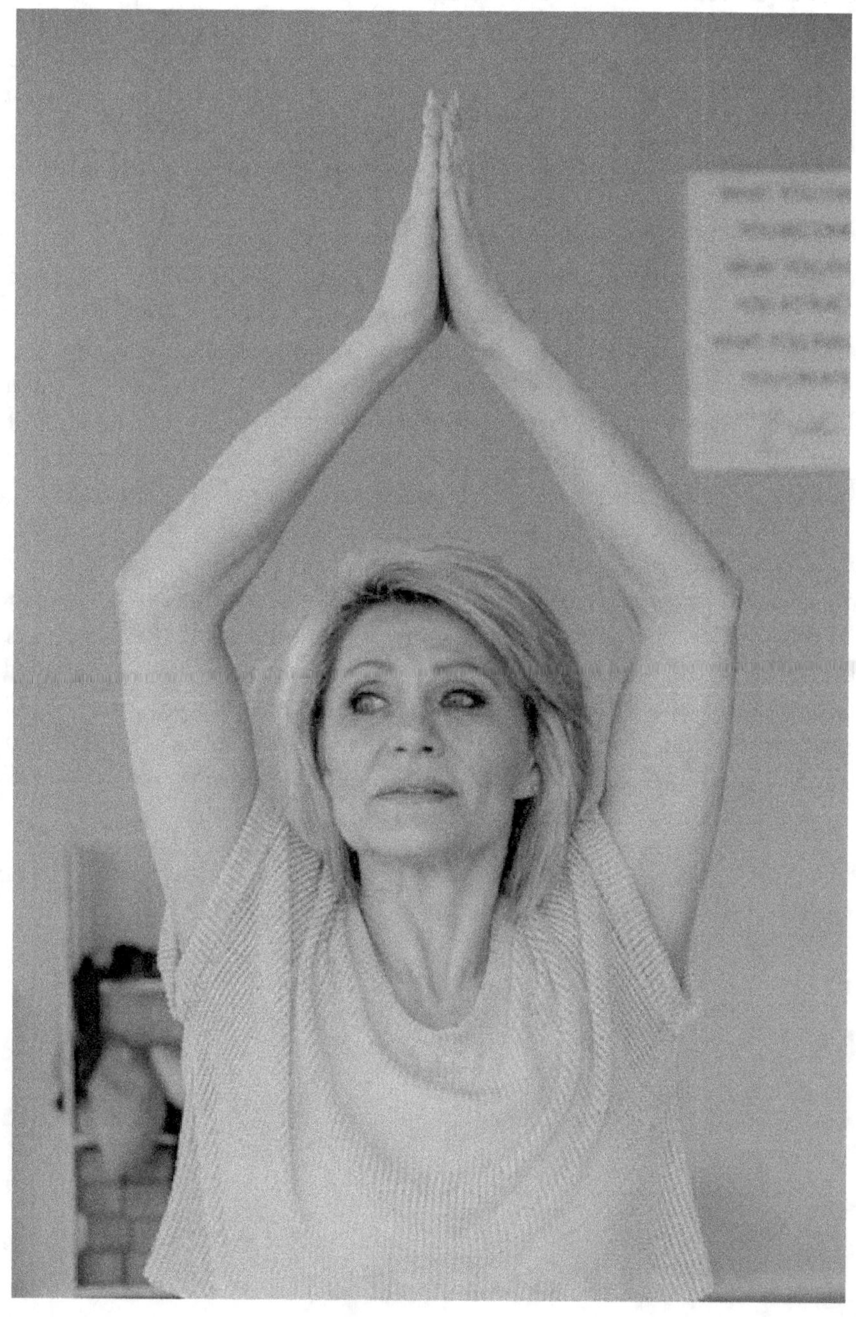

Aging can result in decreased flexibility and increased stiffness, so including regular stretching exercises in your exercise regimen can help with your agility and ability to do your daily chores independently.

Flexibility is a precursor to an active lifestyle, leading to independence and good overall health. Developing flexibility in your muscles makes them strong and helps prevent injury while doing basic actions like lifting, bending, climbing stairs, and exercising. Stretching exercises give your muscles a greater range of motion and allow them to help you carry out physical tasks without the risk of sprains and fractures. Such exercises are categorized as dynamic and static based on the way they are performed.

Dynamic Stretches

Dynamic stretches are not held for an extended period. They are performed rhythmically to increase blood flow, raise body temperature, and decrease muscle stiffness. Because of this, dynamic stretches are good for warm-ups (Bramble, 2021).

In this section, we'll look at some dynamic stretches you can perform to strengthen your muscles.

Shoulder Rolls

1. Sit on your chair, keeping your spine straight.

2. Extend your arms out to each side.

3. Bend your elbows to bring your fingertips to your shoulders.

4. Roll your shoulders in a forward motion 5–10 times.

5. Reverse the direction and roll your shoulders backward 5–10 times.

6. Keep your elbows bent and fingertips touching your shoulders throughout the exercise.

Benefits:

- Seated shoulder rolls help improve joint mobility and flexibility in the shoulders.

- Performing this exercise regularly can help release tension and stiffness in the muscles surrounding the shoulders and upper back, promoting relaxation and reducing discomfort.

- This exercise can help improve posture.

Finger Stretches

This exercise is also called the grip exercise by strength training practitioners.

1. Sit on the chair with your spine upright and feet resting on the ground.

2. Breathe deeply yet gently.

3. Extend your arms forward.

4. Stretch your fingers out and separate them.

5. Clench your hands to make a fist for 5 seconds.

6. Open the fist and spread the fingers again.

7. Repeat 5–10 times.

Benefits:

- This exercise works your hand flexors, extensors, and intrinsic hand muscles.

- It relieves stiffness and improves flexibility in the fingers and hands.

- It reduces the risk of developing health issues like carpal tunnel syndrome and arthritis.

- Finger stretches promote relaxation and reduce tension in the hands, which can benefit overall hand function.

Seated Toe Stretches

1. As you sit on your chair, start deep breathing and coordinate it with your movements during this exercise.

2. Lift your right foot slightly above the ground and stretch your toe muscles by moving them upward, downward, clockwise, and counterclockwise.

3. Return your right foot to the ground and repeat the exercise with your left foot.

Benefits:

- This exercise increases the flexibility in your toes and feet.

- It helps prevent and alleviate foot problems such as plantar fasciitis and bunions.

- The exercise promotes better balance and stability.

Seated Neck Stretches

1. Sit with your back straight, palms resting on your thighs.

2. Inhale deeply as you straighten and extend your neck. Hold for a moment then exhale as you relax the stretch.

3. Inhale deeply again as you tilt your head to the right, hold for a moment, then exhale as you return to center.

4.   Repeat the motions and breathing pattern as you stretch to the left.

Benefits:

- Neck stretches relieve tension and tightness in the neck and shoulders.

- This exercise increases mobility in your neck.

- Neck stretches reduce neck pain and headaches.

Chin-to-Chest Stretch

1.   Sit upright on your chair with good posture.

2.   Inhale as you bring your chin toward your chest, stretching the back of your neck.

3.   Look back up and return your chin to its normal position.

4.   Repeat the motion 8–10 times.

Benefits:

- This stretch can help alleviate tension and improve flexibility in your upper back and neck.

- It can help enhance your posture.

- This stretch can be done throughout the day to help relieve neck stiffness from long periods spent on the computer.

Static Stretches

Static stretches involve holding a position to tighten your muscles and engage your joints by stretching your muscles to the maximum comfortable distance and are good for incorporating into your cool-down session. Static stretches are typically held for no more than 45 seconds, and the duration should be based on the individual's capacity to hold the stretch (Bramble, 2021). A 10–15 second hold is suitable for most seniors.

In this section, we'll explore some static stretches you can add to your workout routine.

Arm Stretches

1. Sit upright with your back straight on your chair.

2. Inhale deeply and exhale.

3. Inhale again as you extend your arms forward, palms facing up and elbows straight. Extend your reach to feel a good stretch.

4. Hold the pose for 5 counts.

5. Bend your elbows to touch your shoulders with your fingertips and hold for a moment.

6. Straighten your arms back out in front of you, resuming the stretch.

7. Perform the exercise 8–10 times.

Benefits:

- Arm stretches improve the mobility of your biceps, triceps, forearms, and deltoids.

- They release tension and stiffness in the arms and shoulders.

- This exercise increases flexibility and mobility in the upper body.

- It enhances blood circulation to the arms, promoting better nutrient delivery and waste removal.

Seated Shoulder Stretch

1. Maintain an upright posture as you sit on your chair.

2. Reach your right arm across your chest at shoulder height.

3. Use your left hand to gently press your right arm into your chest. You should feel a stretch in the upper back and shoulder area on your right side.

4. Hold the stretch for a few breaths, then release.

5. Perform the stretch on the other side by bringing your left arm across your chest and using your right hand to press it gently into your chest.

6. Repeat the exercise 2–4 times with each arm.

Benefits:

- Seated shoulder stretches engage and tone the three shoulder muscles— deltoids, trapezius, and rhomboids.

- This exercise relieves tension and tightness in the upper back and shoulders.

- It helps prevent shoulder injuries and promotes better posture.

Leg Extensions on a Chair

1. Sit up straight on your chair with your feet resting on the ground and your hands holding the chair.

2. Inhale deeply and exhale.

3. Inhale again, and as you exhale, slowly lift your right leg off the ground, extending it forward while keeping it as straight as is comfortable.

4. Hold for a count of 5.

5. Return your right foot to the floor as you exhale.

6. Repeat the stretch with your left leg.

7. Repeat the exercise 5 times on each side.

Benefits:

- Leg extensions engage and strengthen the quadriceps, hamstrings, glutes, and calf muscles.

- They improve stability and balance.

- This stretch enhances circulation in the lower limbs, reducing the risk of blood clots and improving overall leg health.

Forward Fold on a Chair (Paschimottanasana)

1. For this exercise, you may choose to use yoga blocks if you find it hard to bend enough to touch the ground. Place them on the ground before beginning the exercise.

2. Sit on the edge of your chair with your feet resting on the ground hip-width apart.

3. Breathe in deeply and straighten your spine.

4. Exhale gently while reaching your fingertips toward your feet, the ground, or yoga blocks.

5. Try to keep your back as flat as possible.

6. Inhale gently as you straighten back up to an upright position.

Benefits:

- The forward fold exercise stretches the spine, hamstrings, and shoulders.

- It provides relaxation and releases tension in the spine, shoulder, and thighs.

Seated Eagle

1. Sit comfortably on your chair with your feet flat on the floor.

2. Cross your right thigh over your left thigh, and, if possible, wrap your right foot around your left calf.

3. Cross your left arm over your right arm, and if possible, bring your palms together.

4. Hold this position for a few breaths, then release and switch sides.

Benefits:

- The seated eagle stretch improves balance and concentration.

- It stretches the shoulders and upper back.

- This exercise relieves tension in the arms and wrists.

Chair Pigeon Pose

1.   Sit on your chair in an upright position.

2.   Plant your left foot firmly on the ground and cross your right ankle over your left knee.

You can place a firm cushion under your left thigh to support the left knee bearing the extra weight.

3.   Keeping your back straight, apply some gentle pressure on your right knee, pressing it down.

4.   Hold the stretch for a count of 5–10 and then repeat the exercise with your left ankle crossed over your right knee.

Benefits:

- This exercise stretches the outer hip and glute muscles.

- Pigeon pose improves the range of motion in the hip joints and reduces hip stiffness.

- This exercise can help relieve discomfort associated with sciatica.

Techniques for Safe and Effective Stretching

The best exercise session is done safely and should not cause you any pain. Let's talk about some techniques you can practice to get the most out of your workouts (*Six Tips for Safe Stretches*, 2019):

- **Use a stable chair:** Ensure that the chair you use for exercising is sturdy enough to support your weight safely. Opt for an armless chair to allow for a wider range of movement during exercises. Do not use a chair with wheels. Additionally, choose a chair with a backrest to provide support and maintain proper posture throughout your workout.

- **Start with a warm-up session:** Incorporate gentle stretches and rotations into the beginning of your routine to engage your joints and muscles and get them warm to prepare them for exercise and reduce the risk of injury.

- **Remember to breathe:** Hold the stretch but not your breath! Keep breathing gently and deeply to enhance focus and reduce stress.

- **Perform painless stretches:** Move slowly and gently and focus on flexibility and range of motion without pushing past comfort. Pay attention to any discomfort or pain while you're exercising. Adjust your intensity or number of repetitions to prevent strain and injury.

- **Stay committed:** Exercise daily and stay consistent with your routine to reap the full benefits of improved health and fitness over time.

- **Stay hydrated:** Drink water before, during, and after your exercise session to maintain proper hydration levels and support optimal performance and recovery.

Incorporating flexibility training or stretching exercises into your overall fitness regimen is important to lay the groundwork for strength training. Stretching exercises optimize your overall muscular performance by elongating the muscle fibers and increasing the blood flow. Strength training, which involves progressively overloading muscles with resistance, is the next step for building muscle strength. Incorporating strength training into your yoga routines can stimulate the production of muscle fibers and support bone health. Now that you have some tools for increasing your flexibility, let's transition to the next chapter to learn how you can increase your physical capabilities with strength training exercises.

Chapter 3:

Discover the Strength in Sitting

You have to push past your perceived limits, push past that point you thought was as far as you can go. –Drew Brees

As a beginner, practicing various poses ranging from stretches to foundational postures like seated poses and gentle twists can help you build strength, flexibility, and body awareness. Once you get into the habit of exercising regularly, you will begin to strengthen your major muscle groups, such as your core, back, arm, and leg muscles (Pizer, 2018). Gradually introducing more challenging poses as you progress can foster continuous growth and improvement in your practice. Yoga also has a positive effect on your mental health as you may begin to feel more calm and focused.

Yoga is a diverse discipline of exercise. There are yoga exercises that make your body work against your body weight, such as plank pose, four-limbed staff pose, and arm balances like crow pose or cobra pose. These poses require you to engage muscles to support and stabilize your body, building strength and endurance.

Integrating other types of exercise with yoga promotes diversity in movement patterns, which can help prevent overuse injuries and promote balanced muscle development. Doing strength training exercises such as weight lifting or body-weight exercises alongside yoga can enhance muscular strength and endurance, supporting stability and alignment in yoga postures (*Why It's Good*, n.d.). Strength training can make your bones stronger, build up your muscles, and lower the risk of fractures and osteoporosis as you age.

What Is Strength Training?

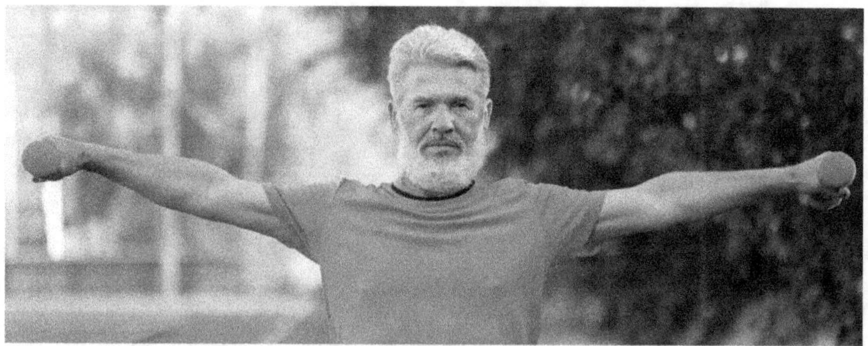

Strength training, also known as weight training or resistance training, is a form of exercise that makes you work against your body weight or an external weight to make you stronger (Seguin & Nelson, 2003). These exercises put stress on your muscles and bones. In response, your muscles adapt by repairing and growing bigger muscle fibers, and new bone cells are formed. These kinds of exercises also work your joints and increase blood flow and synovial fluid circulation.

Strength Training Exercises With Body Weight

Examples of body-weight exercises on a chair include wall push-ups, seated leg raises, chair lunges, and seated knee lifts. With these exercises, your muscles have to work against the weight of your body.

Seated Wall Push-Ups

1. Sit on a chair facing a wall about an arm's distance from the wall.

2. Place your palms at a comfortable distance apart on the wall.

3. Bend your elbows and apply gentle pressure on the wall with both palms.

4. As you apply pressure, bend your elbows to ease your upper body toward the wall.

5. Pause for a moment then gently straighten your elbows to push your upper body back to the starting position.

6. Repeat 4–5 times.

Benefits:

- This simple exercise boosts strength in your chest, shoulders, and arms.

- Wall push-ups improve upper body stability and posture.

Seated Knee Lifts

1. With your back straight and feet resting on the floor, sit on the edge of your chair.

2. Stabilize yourself by holding the sides of the seat of the chair.

3. Lift your right knee and bring it toward your chest. Keep your shoulders relaxed throughout the exercise.

4. Hold for a moment then lower your right knee back down to the starting position.

5. Repeat the movement using your left leg.

6. Perform 5–10 repetitions with each leg.

Benefits:

- Knee lifts improve core strength and stability.

- This exercise helps in maintaining balance and coordination.

Chair Lunges

1. Take your seat and get ready for the exercise by keeping your back straight and feet flat on the floor at a comfortable distance from one another.

2. Shift your weight slightly forward toward the edge of the chair.

3. Grip the sides of the chair firmly for support and stability.

4. Lift your hips slightly off the chair.

5. Slide one foot forward, bending the knee and lowering your hips toward the floor while keeping your back straight.

6. Use your legs to push yourself back to the starting position.

7. Repeat the exercise with the other leg.

8. Perform 5–10 repetitions on each leg.

Benefits:

- Chair lunges boost strength in the quadricep, hamstring, and glute muscles.

- They strengthen your lower body, improving your stability and balance.

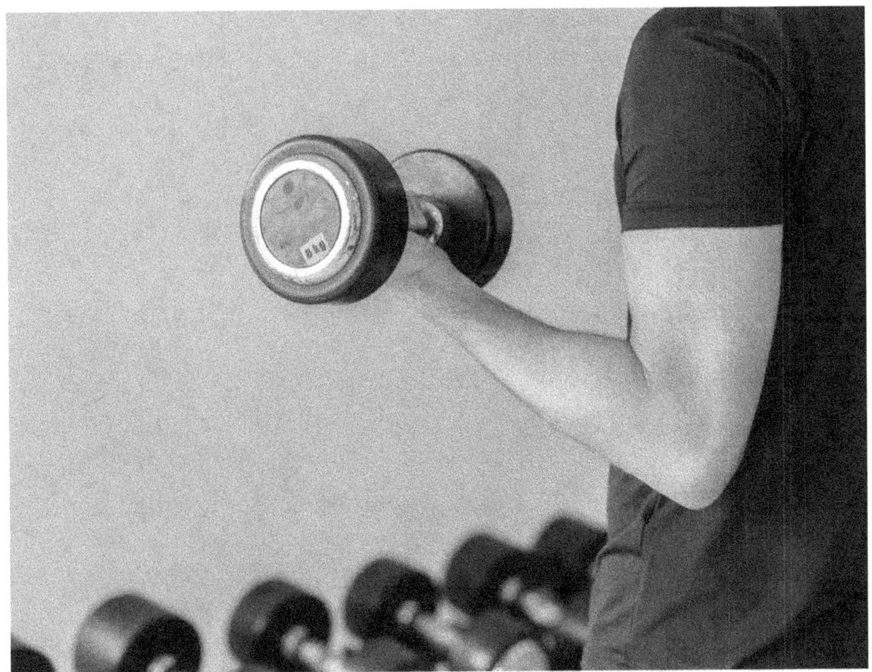

Once you have learned to use your body weight to develop muscle and bone mass, you can start incorporating resistance bands and light weights while sitting comfortably. External weights and resistance bands help shape and build your muscles and make your bones strong and healthy. Using external weights or resistance bands allows you to target and tone specific muscle groups. For example, you may lift 3–5 lb. dumbbells to strengthen your arm muscles and use a resistance band to tone up your leg muscles.

Bicep Curls

1. Sit upright on your chair, keeping your feet flat and hip-width apart.

2. Hold dumbbells in both hands with your arms straight down and palms facing upward.

3. Keeping your elbows close to your sides, bend them slowly to lift the dumbbells toward your shoulders.

4. Slowly straighten your arms to return the dumbbells back to the starting position.

5. Repeat 5-10 times.

Benefits:

- Bicep curls increase arm strength.

- This strength training exercise improves muscle tone and definition in the arms.

- It helps in performing daily activities requiring arm strength.

Tricep Curls

1. Sit upright on your chair keeping your feet firmly on the ground at a comfortable distance from each other.

2. With a dumbbell in your right hand, extend your arm at a comfortable angle behind you to engage the tricep muscles located at the back of your upper arm.

3. Raise your forearm gently to bring the weight toward your shoulder while keeping the upper arm stationary.

4. Keep your left hand at rest on the chair's edge.

5. Bend your elbow, lowering the dumbbell to the starting position.

6. Perform 5–10 repetitions then switch to the other arm.

Benefits:

- Tricep curls focus on the triceps muscles, aiding in arm extension.

- The exercise helps tone and sculpt the back of the arms.

- It improves overall arm strength.

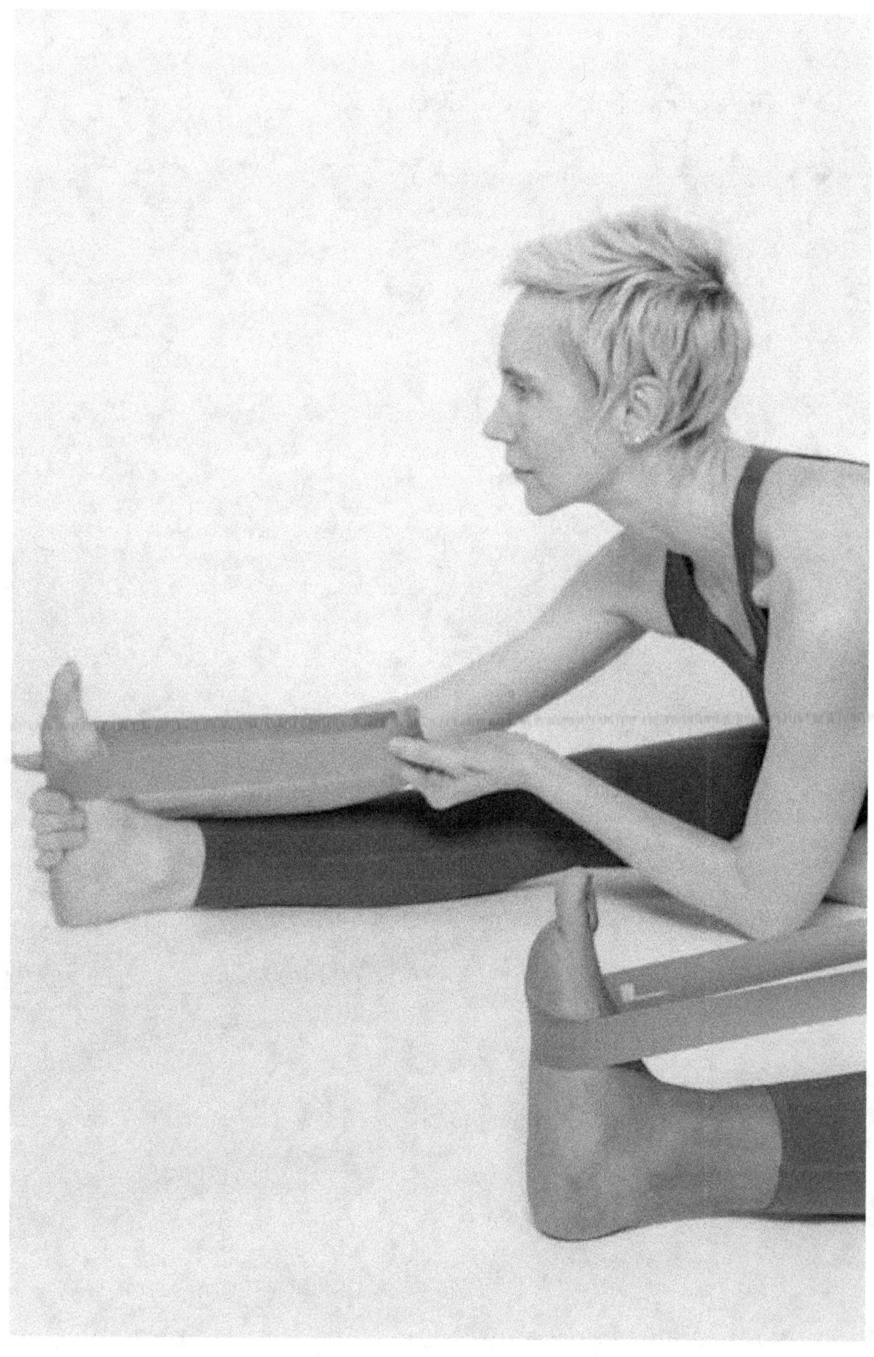

Seated resistance band exercises offer a convenient and effective alternative for individuals with mobility issues or limitations. A resistance band is an elastic band that provides resistance during various forms of exercise. It also provides comfort in performing exercises by offering a cushioned and flexible grip, which can reduce strain on your hands and wrists during workouts. Exercises such as squats, chest presses, and seated rows are easier to perform while seated on a chair and using a resistance band than their traditional forms.

Squats With a Chair

1. Stand in front of your chair with your feet shoulder-width apart.

2. Lower your body by bending your knees and hips as if you were about to sit. Keep your chest upright and your weight in your heels.

3. Use the chair for support as needed and remember to breathe.

4. Apply some pressure on your heels to stand back up to the starting position.

5. Repeat 5–10 times.

Benefits:

- Squats strengthen your quadriceps, hamstrings, and glutes, improving the functional fitness of your lower body.

- They enable your legs to support your weight.

Seated Chest Presses

1. Get ready for this exercise by sitting upright on your chair.

2. Hold a dumbbell in each hand at chest height with your elbows bent.

3. Press the dumbbells straight out in front of you until your arms are fully extended.

4. Slowly bend your elbows to bring your hands back to the sides of your chest.

5. Repeat 3–5 times, increasing the number of repetitions over time.

Benefits:

- Chest presses strengthen your chest muscles.

- They make the shoulder and arm muscles stronger.

- This exercise tones your upper body muscles.

Seated Rows With a Resistance Band

1. Sit up straight on your chair.

2. Step on the resistance band with both feet, keeping your feet firmly on the ground.

3. Hold the ends of the resistance band in each hand with your arms extended in front of you.

4. Pull the resistance band toward yourself, bringing your shoulder blades together.

5. Slowly return to the starting position.

6. Repeat 3–5 times, increasing the number of repetitions over time.

Benefits:

- Seated rows work on the rhomboids and trapezius muscles in the upper back.

- This exercise helps improve posture by strengthening the muscles responsible for shoulder blade retraction.

- They enhance back strength and stability.

Muscle-Strengthening Yoga Exercises

Yoga exercises that strengthen your muscles are indeed body-weight exercises. While the results may become apparent more gradually, starting your strength training journey with yoga is safe and effective. It helps build muscular endurance, improve stability, and enhance overall functional strength. Additionally, yoga enables you to practice lifting external weights without the risk of injury by emphasizing proper alignment, mindful movement, and controlled breathing, which all contribute to a safer and more sustainable approach to strength building.

Supine Boat Pose (Ardha Navasana)

1. Lie flat on your back on your bed with your legs extended.

2. On an inhale, lift your legs off the bed, keeping them together with your knees bent, aiming for a 45-degree angle from the bed's surface.

3. Extend your arms forward, keeping them parallel to the bed with your fingers pointing toward your toes.

4. Engage your abdominal muscles to lift your upper body slightly while extending your hands.

5. Balance on your sit bones while using your legs and torso to balance and create a V shape.

6. Extend your arms parallel to your legs while trying to reach for your toes.

7. Hold the pose for several breaths, keeping your chest lifted and your gaze focused on your toes.

8. Exhale while gradually lowering your legs and arms back to the starting position.

9. Rest for a moment, allowing your body to relax.

10. Repeat the supine boat pose 2–4 times, gradually increasing the duration of the hold.

Benefits:

- Supine boat pose helps make your core resilient.

- This exercise strengthens the leg muscles.

- It makes the spine more flexible.

- Supine boat pose stimulates digestion.

- This exercise helps improve posture.

Prone Boat Pose (Naukasana)

1. Lie flat on your stomach with your legs extended and your arms resting alongside your body, palms facing down.

2. Draw your navel toward your spine to engage your core muscles.

3. Inhale and gently lift your chest and legs off the bed simultaneously. Keep your gaze forward and avoid straining your neck by keeping it in a neutral position.

4. As you lift your chest and legs, extend your arms forward, reaching your fingertips out in front of you. Your arms should be parallel to the ground with your palms facing each other.

5. Press through your heels and lift your thighs off the bed to engage your leg muscles. Aim to keep your legs straight and active throughout the pose.

6. Hold the pose for several breaths, maintaining steady breathing. Keep your core engaged to support your lower back and continue to lift through your chest and legs.

7. Exhale as you gently lower your chest and legs back down to the bed. Rest for a moment in the starting position, allowing your body to relax.

8. You can repeat the prone boat pose several times, gradually increasing the duration of the hold as you build strength and endurance.

Benefits:
- Prone boat pose strengthens the core muscles and spine.

- It strengthens your back.

- The exercise tones the leg muscles.

- It helps you become more aware of your body's position and movements. This awareness is called proprioception.

- Prone boat pose stimulates digestion and enhances blood circulation.

- It refreshes you mentally and physically.

Plank Pose (Phalakasana)

1. Start on your bed in a push-up position, keeping your palms on the bed directly under your shoulders with your body making a straight line from your head to your heels.

2. Press your palms and toes firmly into the bed.

3. Hold the position for 10 seconds, aiming to maintain a straight back with proper alignment and stability throughout.

4. To release, gently lower your knees to the bed and rest in child's pose or transition to another pose.

Benefits:

- Plank pose strengthens your core muscles.

- It makes your shoulders, arms, and chest stronger when performed regularly.

- This exercise improves spinal alignment and stability.

- It enhances balance and stability through the engagement of the entire body.

- Plank pose boosts the strength of the spinal and pelvis muscles.

Four-Limbed Staff Pose (Chaturanga Dandasana)

This is a modified version of the classic plank pose explained above.

1. Lie on your stomach on your bed.

2. Separate your legs slightly and keep your knees straight.

3. Place your palms on the bed near your ribcage, fingers spread wide and pointing forward.

4. Tighten your core muscles to offer support to your lower back.

5. Inhale and press into your palms, lifting your chest and upper body off the bed. Keep your elbows close to your sides, bent and pointing backward, and engage your shoulder blades by drawing them down and back.

6. To make this pose more accessible, keep your knees on the bed. This reduces the amount of weight your upper body has to support and makes it easier to maintain proper alignment.

7. If lifting the chest and upper body is challenging, you can also keep your forearms on the bed with your elbows bent at a 90-degree angle.

8. Hold the pose for 5–10 counts, then slowly lower your upper body back down to the starting position.

9. Focus on breathing deeply and evenly while holding this pose.

Benefits:

- This exercise supports and strengthens the upper and lower back muscles and the abdomen.

- The four-limbed staff pose increases flexibility in the spine and chest through gentle backbend stretches.

- The pose stimulates circulation throughout the body, delivering oxygen and nutrients to muscles and organs and boosting mood and energy levels.

- It helps improve posture.

Cobra Pose on Bed (Bhujangasana)

1. Lie on your stomach on the bed with your palms placed flat on the mattress near your ribcage.

2. Inhale and gently press into your palms and lift your chest and head off the bed. Focus on using your back muscles rather than your arms to lift your head and chest.

3. Keep your elbows near your sides to target your back muscles. Keep your shoulders down and your gaze forward, curving your back inward.

4. Maintain the pose for a count of 5–10, then exhale and come back to the original lying position.

Benefits:

- Cobra pose stretches the spine and chest muscles.

- It adds strength to your back muscles and reduces back pain.

- This stretch enhances your posture.

Chair Crow Pose (Bakasana)

1. Sit on your chair without using the backrest for support.

2. Bend your knees at a 90-degree angle.

3. Place two yoga blocks on the ground in front of the chair a few inches away.

4. Lean forward and hold the yoga blocks firmly with your hands.

5. With your feet firmly on the ground, lift your hips slightly off the chair, transferring your weight to your hands and arms.

6. Lift your right foot off the ground while bringing your chest toward your knees.

7. Hold for a count of 5–10, then come back to the sitting position.

8. Repeat the exercise with your left foot.

9. During this pose, balance and support your weight with your hands and arms, maintaining a strong core and steady breath.

10. Rest for a moment before doing another set of this exercise.

Benefits:

- Crow pose boosts strength in your arm, shoulder, and core muscles.

- It improves balance and proprioception.

- This exercise engages the muscles of the upper body and abdomen.

- It enhances focus and concentration.

- Crow pose offers a gentle introduction to arm balance exercises for beginners or individuals with wrist issues.

The strength training exercises mentioned in this chapter can help reverse the effects of aging by strengthening your muscles and bones and preventing injuries, sprains, and fractures. Remember to take all safety measures like using 3–5 lb. dumbbells, incorporating deep breathing while exercising, keeping yourself hydrated, having a light meal an hour before exercising, and taking breaks between exercises to keep your heart rate in check.

The heart is a muscle too, and strengthening and energizing it is crucial for maintaining overall health and vitality. In the next chapter, we'll talk about how you can integrate yoga and cardio to be heart-healthy.

Chapter 4:

Combine Chair Cardio and Yoga to Energize Your Heart

Do your part, care for your heart. –Unknown

Your heart, blood vessels, blood, and plasma make up your circulatory system, or the cardiovascular system. Regular exercise can benefit your cardiovascular health even more when paired with a low-calorie, high-nutrient diet. Exercise lowers the risk of developing heart diseases by burning excess calories, lowering your blood pressure, reducing inflammation, reducing the secretion of stress hormones, and energizing the heart. If you are wondering how exercise energizes your heart, let me explain! Exercise increases the heart rate, improving its ability to pull more oxygen from the purified blood supplied by the lungs. So when the heart beats faster, it has to work less, leading to less stress (*Exercise and the Heart*, n.d.).

Even mimicking the motions of cardio activities like walking, cycling, swimming, and dancing while seated can offer advantages to your muscles and joints. This innovative approach can improve your fitness if you have mobility constraints or seek gentler forms of exercise to reduce stress on the body. Simple cardio exercises done regularly at home, even without specialized equipment, are effective and safe for seniors.

Advantages of Seated Cardio Exercises

Here's how simple cardiovascular exercises done in the comfort of your chair benefit your body:

- **Heart health:** Cardiovascular exercises strengthen the heart muscle, improving its efficiency in pumping blood throughout the body. This helps your heart function well.

- **Holistic health:** By increasing blood flow, these exercises enhance blood circulation, delivering oxygen and nutrients to tissues and organs while removing waste and toxins. This promotes better overall health and function of the body's systems.

- **Lung health:** Cardio exercises involve rhythmic, repetitive movements that require increased oxygen intake. This helps expand lung capacity and improves respiratory efficiency, enhancing oxygen delivery to the bloodstream.

- **Weight management:** Burning calories and reducing body fat can be made possible by consistent practice of cardio exercises.

- **Enhanced endurance:** You can boost your energy and stamina and increase your body's ability to sustain physical activity without becoming fatigued when you incorporate seated cardio into your exercise routine.

- **Stress reduction:** A cardio session can stimulate the release of endorphins, which are neurotransmitters that promote feelings of well-being and reduce stress and anxiety.

- **Improved metabolic health:** You can regulate your blood sugar levels, improve insulin sensitivity, and lower cholesterol levels with cardio exercise, reducing the risk of metabolic disorders such as diabetes and metabolic syndrome.

The heart health benefits to be gained from seated cardiovascular exercises are comparable to the benefits offered by traditional cardio exercises. Chair-based cardio workouts are low-impact and accessible to individuals with lower mobility or other health concerns.

Combining Yoga and Cardio

Practicing yoga helps you exercise different muscle groups and build muscular awareness, while cardio is good for improving respiratory health, lowering stress and blood pressure, and losing weight. Incorporating cardio into your yoga regimen can help you derive more holistic benefits and take your exercise journey to new levels. For instance, the respiratory benefits from yogic deep breathing can be improved even more if you include cardio exercises. Yoga helps reduce stress, and when done in conjunction with cardio, your improved lung capacity and heart rate can strengthen the stress control mechanism of your body (The Man Flow Yoga Team, n.d.).

Seated cardio exercises can increase your heart rate, so starting and ending your exercise session with a gentle yoga warm-up and cool-down session is recommended for getting the most out of your workout (SarahBethYoga, 2022).

Precautions to Take Before Practicing Seated Cardio

To make your chair exercise session fun, there are a few things to keep in mind:

- **Take medical advice:** Before beginning cardio exercises, consult your doctor, especially if you have any pre-existing health conditions.

- **Do not start your exercise routine with cardio exercises:** Because cardio workouts increase your heart rate, start with mild yoga stretches and deep breathing to get your heart and mind into the flow gradually.

- **Practice mild cardio:** Practice mild seated cardio exercises like seated marching, seated swimming, and seated cycling. Knowing your abilities and limits and not feeling pressure to get results quickly ensures safety while exercising.

- **Relax your body and mind:** Pranayama, or relaxing yoga poses like corpse pose, child's pose, or legs up the wall pose, help you ease the stress on your muscles, joints, and mind and provide relaxation.

So ensure you have taken all necessary precautions and get ready to increase your heart rate with fun and vibrant seated cardio exercises to revitalize your cardiovascular system and enhance your energy levels.

Fun Seated Cardio Exercises

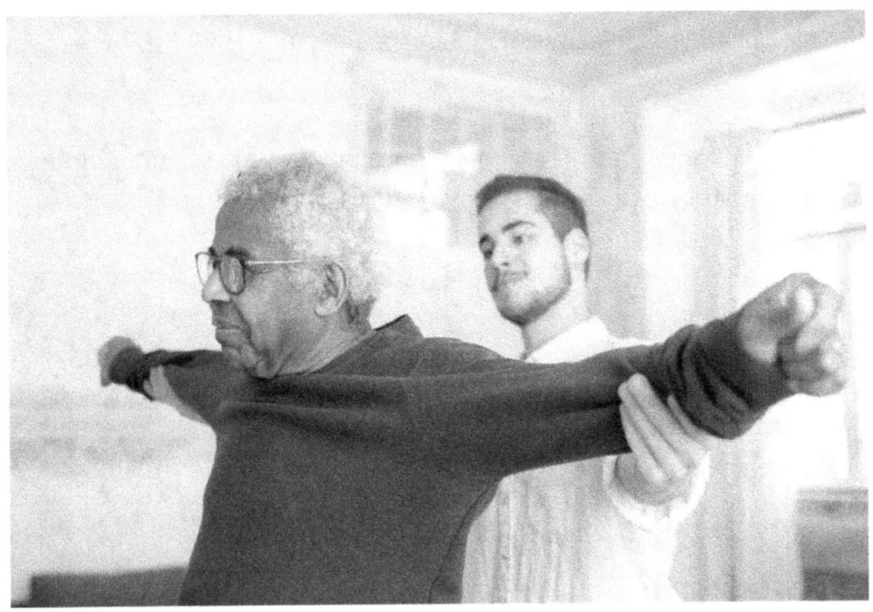

If you have difficulty walking long distances, consider strolling with support within your own home. Exercises such as seated walking, marching, swimming, and cycling can help improve your mobility. Modifying these activities provides similar benefits as doing the traditional versions because you are addressing the same muscles and joints from the comfort of your chair.

Seated Walking

1.   Sit on your chair in a comfortable position, breathing steadily and holding the sides of the chair with both hands.

2.   Lift your right leg up off the floor, keeping your knee bent and back straight.

3.   Return your right leg to the ground and repeat the motion with your left leg.

4. Repeat 10 times with each leg.

Benefits:

- Seated walking improves blood circulation and cardiovascular health.

- This exercise helps maintain joint mobility and range of motion, particularly in the hips and knees.

- It boosts leg strength by engaging the quadriceps, hamstrings, and calf muscles.

- Seated walking can be performed anywhere, making it suitable for individuals with limited mobility or those undergoing rehabilitation.

Seated Marching

1. Breathe gently and deeply as you sit on your chair.

2. Lift your right leg up off the floor and pump your left arm forward and your right arm backward, keeping your elbows bent.

3. Return your right leg to the ground and lift your left leg up, pumping your right arm forward and your left arm backward.

4. Repeat 10 times with each leg.

Benefits:

- Seated marching enhances coordination and balance.

- It engages core muscles, including the abdominals and lower back, for improved stability.

- This exercise increases heart rate and calorie expenditure, promoting cardiovascular fitness.

Seated Freestyle Swimming

1. Sit up straight on your chair, breathing gently and deeply.

2. Swing your arms back and forth and gently rotate your shoulders to prepare your muscles for the exercise.

3. Pretend to swim in freestyle by alternating reaching your arms out in front of you and moving them in a circular motion.

4. While performing the arm movements, lift your legs slightly above the ground and kick them downward.

5. Repeat 10 times.

Benefits:
- Seated freestyle swimming offers a full-body workout, engaging muscles from head to toe.

- This exercise improves cardiovascular endurance.

- It alleviates stress on joints, making it ideal for individuals with arthritis or joint pain.

Seated High Knee Raises

1. Sit up straight slightly away from the chair's backrest.

2. Take deep gentle breaths and hold the sides of your chair for support.

3. Keeping your upper body straight, lift one knee toward your chest as high as you comfortably can.

4. Lower the leg and lift the other knee toward your chest.

5. Alternate lifting knees as quickly as possible while maintaining good posture.

6. Repeat 8–10 times with each leg.

Benefits:

- Seated high knee raises increase your heart rate and improve cardiovascular health.

- They boost strength in your quadriceps and hip flexors.

- This exercise enhances core stability and balance.

- It flexes your hip joints.

- Seated high knee raises boost circulation and promote blood flow throughout the body.

Side Leg Tap

1. With your hands on your waist, sit upright in your chair.

2. Inhale deeply then lift one leg and extend it out to the side, keeping your back straight.

3. When your leg reaches its furthest point to the side, lightly tap the ground with your toes.

4. Return your leg to the starting position and repeat the same action with the other leg.

5. Alternate side leg taps 8–10 times on each side.

Benefits:

- Side leg taps strengthen and tone the muscles in the legs, including the hips, thighs, and glutes.

- They improve balance and stability by engaging core muscles and requiring coordination to perform the movement while seated.

- They enhance flexibility in the hip joints and improve the range of motion of the legs.

- This exercise helps reduce stiffness and discomfort that can result from sitting for long durations.

Side Arm Cardio

1. Sit upright on your chair.

2. Keep your feet a comfortable distance apart.

3. Rest your palms on the chair by your sides.

4. Extend your right arm diagonally in front of you, then return it to the starting position.

5. Repeat the same with your left arm.

6. Alternate between arms in a quick and controlled manner, engaging your arm muscles throughout the exercise.

7. Repeat 8–10 times with each arm.

Benefits:

- The side arm cardio exercise strengthens the muscles in the arms, including the shoulders, biceps, and triceps.

- This exercise improves motor skills.

- It increases your heart rate and provides a cardiovascular workout when performed at a fast pace.

- Side arm cardio tones and sculpts the arms, contributing to overall muscle definition.

- This exercise can be easily modified to suit different fitness levels by adjusting the speed and intensity of the movements.

- It is convenient to perform this exercise anywhere, making it a versatile exercise option for home, office, or travel.

Seated Cardio to Boost Your Energy and Stamina

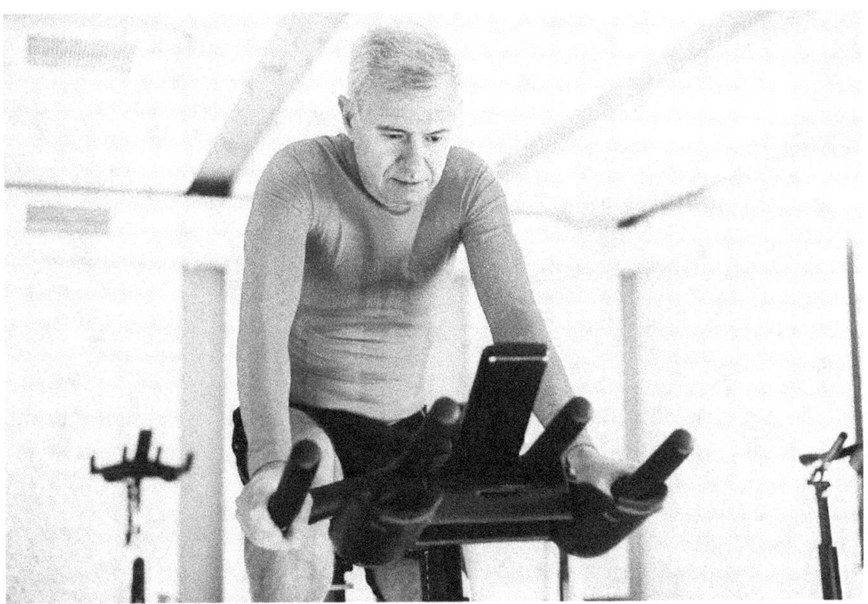

In this section, we'll look at some invigorating seated cardio exercises designed to enhance energy levels and stamina.

Seated Bicycle Crunches

1. Sit on a chair with your back straight and feet flat on the floor.

2. Pointing your elbows in opposite directions, place your hands lightly behind your head.

3. Bring your right knee toward your chest while bringing your left elbow to touch the right knee. Twist through your torso to reach your elbow to your knee.

4. Return to the starting position and repeat the exercise with your left knee and right elbow.

5. Control your breathing and engage your core muscles while performing this exercise.

6. Do 6–8 repetitions on each side.

Benefits:

- Bicycle crunches provide a low-impact cardiovascular workout.

- This exercise lessens the pressure on the joints.

Tip:

1. Use a stationary bike for cycling practice if it's convenient and comfortable.

2. Take precautions such as adjusting the seat height to ensure proper alignment and consulting with a healthcare professional or fitness expert for guidance on suitable intensity levels and duration.

Jumping Jacks With Support

1. Stand close to your chair for support.

2. Keep your feet together and your hands resting lightly on the chair's backrest.

3. Step your right foot out to the side.

4. Raise both arms above your head.

5. Return your right foot to the starting position and lower your arms, bringing them back to your sides.

6. Repeat the motion with your left foot, stepping it out to the side while raising your arms overhead.

7. Return to the starting position.

8. Continue to alternate stepping out with each foot while moving your arms up and down.

9. Focus on breathing deeply while doing the exercise.

10. If you feel unsteady or uncomfortable, reduce the range of motion or slow down the pace.

11. Aim to perform 5 repetitions to warm up your body and boost circulation.

Benefits:

- Jumping jacks improve the health of your heart.

- They enhance bone density.

- This exercise increases joint mobility.

- It boosts mood and improves cognitive function.

- Jumping jacks enhance your balance and coordination.

Yoga Exercises That Are Good for Your Heart

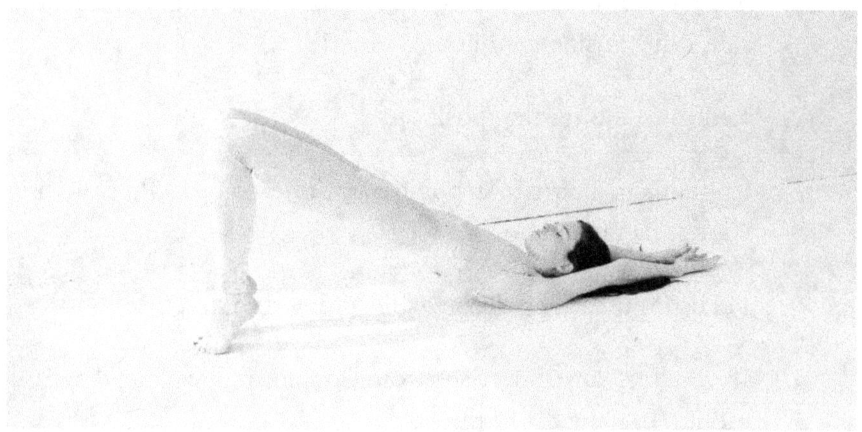

While yoga is not typically considered a high-intensity cardio workout like running, swimming, or cycling, certain yoga sequences and poses can elevate your heart rate and provide cardiovascular benefits. You can modify the standing poses to be performed while seated and perform the lying poses by using a bed instead of a yoga mat on the ground. The goal is to engage the same muscle groups and incorporate deep breathing to benefit your heart health.

As a senior, it is safest to consult your healthcare provider before trying a new kind of exercise. They will recommend safe methods and precautions based on your individual health needs and any pre-existing medical conditions you may have. Let's look at a few exercises that open the chest and improve blood circulation to the heart.

Prone Bow Pose on Bed

1. Lie on your stomach on your bed.

2. Bend your knees and reach backward, trying to grab your ankles.

3. Inhale as you lift your chest and thighs off the bed, creating a bow shape with your body.

4. Hold the pose for 5 counts.

5. Gently release the pose and come back to the original lying position.

Benefits:

- Prone bow pose stretches the front of the body, including the chest, abdomen, and thighs.

- It strengthens your back muscles.

- This exercise improves posture.

- Prone bow pose flexes your spine.

Supine Bow Pose on Bed

1. Lie on your back on the bed with your arms by your sides.

2. Bend your knees to bring your heels toward your hips, resting them flat on the bed.

3. Try to gently grab your ankles with your hands.

4. Inhale as you lift your chest and thighs off the bed, arching your back.

5. Hold the pose for 5 counts.

6. Release the pose and come back to the initial position.

Benefits:

- Supine bow pose stretches the front of the body, including the chest, shoulders, and abdomen.

- This pose strengthens the muscles in your back.

- It improves flexibility and mobility in the spine.

Bridge Pose (Setu Bandhasana)

1. Lie flat on your back on the bed with your knees bent and feet firmly on the mattress.

2. Keep your arms by your sides with the palms facing down.

3. Press your feet into the bed and lift your hips toward the ceiling, engaging your glutes and core muscles.

4. Keep your shoulders relaxed and try to lengthen your spine.

5. Hold the pose for a few breaths, then slowly lower your hips back down to the bed.

6. Repeat the bridge pose 4–5 times, focusing on your breath and maintaining proper form.

Benefits:

- Bridge pose provides a gentle stretch to the spine, hips, and chest muscles.

- This pose opens the chest, stretches the spine, and strengthens the back, buttocks, and thighs.

Fish Pose (Matsyasana)

1. Lie on the bed on your back with your legs extended and arms placed comfortably by your sides.

2. Bend your elbows and place your palms flat on the bed under your hips to support your lower back.

3. Slide your hands as far under your hips as you can with your elbows tucked in close to your body.

4. Press your forearms and elbows firmly into the bed and gently lift your chest and upper back off the bed. Arch your back and lift your heart upward.

5. If comfortable, you can gently tilt your head back and let it rest on the bed, allowing your neck to lengthen. You can use a cushion or pillow for additional support.

6. Hold the pose for a count of 5–10.

7. Gently lower your back, keeping your head back on the bed, and release your arms by your sides.

Benefits:

- Fish pose makes your chest, throat, and abdomen muscles work.

- It stimulates the thyroid gland to work properly.

Seated Sun Salutation (Surya Namaskar)

1. Begin seated on a chair with your feet flat on the floor, your spine tall, and your palms resting on your knees.

2. Inhale gently.

3.   Raise your arms up toward the sky.

4.   Exhale while lowering your arms, folding your torso forward, and bringing your fingers down to the sides of your feet. Try to keep your back as straight as possible.

5.   Sit up straight again.

6.   Repeat this movement 3–5 times, coordinating your breath with your movements.

Benefits:

- Seated sun salutation improves circulation and flexibility.

- It boosts energy and uplifts mood.

- This exercise promotes focus and mental clarity.

Body Mass Index

Your heart health largely depends on your lifestyle. An active routine that involves regular physical activity is crucial to staying heart-healthy and in shape. Equally crucial is the diet you consume. Opting for a diet abundant in nutrients like fiber, antioxidants, and healthy fats is excellent for your heart. Conversely, minimizing your intake of saturated and trans fats, as well as excess salt and sugar, can greatly benefit cardiovascular health. It's all about fueling your body with the right ingredients to keep your heart pumping smoothly.

Body mass index (BMI) measures your body fat based on your weight and height and indicates whether a person has a healthy weight for their height.

Knowing your BMI can be beneficial as it provides context for how you can manage your weight to ensure your cardiovascular fitness. Your BMI is influenced by various factors including diet, exercise, and lifestyle choices. You can compute your BMI and take action accordingly to achieve better health.

BMI is calculated by dividing a person's weight in kilograms by the square of their height in meters. It's a screening tool to indicate whether a person is underweight, normal weight, overweight, or obese (*Calculate Your Body Mass Index*, n.d.).

BMI formula	weight in kilograms ÷ square of height in meters

Avoiding unhealthy fats like saturated and trans fats in your diet and eating more antioxidant-rich foods like nuts, seeds, herbs, fruits, and vegetables can help you manage your BMI. Omega-3 fatty acids aid in reducing inflammation and promoting satiety, while antioxidants support metabolism and cellular health, both of which can positively influence BMI management and contribute to good heart health. Antioxidants, found in fruits, vegetables, nuts, and whole grains, also support heart health.

Here is a chart of the BMI categories (*Calculate Your Body Mass Index*, n.d.):

BMI range	Category
<18.5	Underweight
18.5–24.9	Normal weight
25–29.9	Overweight
30+	Obese

A Cardio + Strength Training Sequence to Burn Calories and Maintain a Healthy BMI

You will need a resistance band to perform this exercise sequence that aims to burn excess calories and tone your muscles. If you are uncomfortable exercising on a mat, do it in the comfort of your bed.

Warm-Up

Start the session with deep breathing. You can also say a prayer or think of the objectives to be achieved for the day. Perform simple stretches like arm stretches, ankle and wrist rotations, and leg extensions before you begin the following sequence.

One: Upper Tummy Exercise

1. Sit on your bed with your legs extended in front of you.

2. Firmly hold the band's ends and wrap the band around the balls of your feet.

3. Lean your body back until you are lying down with your head on the bed, stretching the band. Breathe deeply through the exercise.

4. Come back to the sitting position using your abdominal muscles.

5. Repeat the exercise 3–5 times initially and slowly increase the number of repetitions over a few weeks or months according to your progress.

Two: Lower Tummy Exercise

1. Lie flat on the bed with your legs outstretched.

2. Hold the ends of the resistance band.

3. Flex your feet and pass the band around the balls of your feet.

4. Bring your legs up in the air until they reach a 90-degree angle or as far as is comfortable, keeping the band wrapped around your feet. Hold for a count of 5.

5. Lower your legs back to the bed.

6. Based on your comfort, try to raise and lower your legs without bending at the knees 5–8 times.

Three: Chest and Arms Firming Exercise

1. Sit upright on your bed with your back straight and your legs extended straight out in front of you.

2. Hold the resistance band's ends with your hands and wrap it around the balls of your feet.

3. Keep your hands in line with your shoulders and chest as you curl your hands toward your shoulders and lower them back down.

4. Do 5–10 repetitions.

Four: Hip and Thigh Muscles Toning Exercise

1. Lie flat on your back with your knees bent and feet flat on the bed.

2. Lift your feet and bring your knees toward your chest. Continue breathing throughout the exercise.

3. Hold for a moment before lowering your feet back to the bed again.

4. Repeat this motion 8–10 times.

Cool Down

It is essential to relax your muscles, joints, and brain after a workout. Sitting on your chair, cross your legs, keep your palms on your thighs, close your eyes, and relax with support from the chair's backrest. Breathe deeply for a count of 10.

This exercise sequence will help you burn excess fat, helping to flatten your belly, firm your chest, and tone your arm, hip, and thigh muscles. When performed consistently, it can help you manage your weight and keep your heart healthy.

It's imperative to recognize the interconnectedness of our body's systems. Just as the heart serves as the lifeline of our cardiovascular health, our spinal column stands as the cornerstone of our structural integrity. In the next chapter, we'll look at the role a resilient and well-aligned spine plays in your life and how to keep it strong.

Chapter 5:

Spine-Strengthening Yoga Exercises

The spine is the lifeline. A lot of people should go to a chiropractor but they don't know it. –Jack LaLanne

Your spine supports your body and makes movement possible. It consists of 24 small bones called vertebrae that are stacked on top of each other. There are gel-like disks between each vertebra that act as shock absorbers and keep the bones safe from external pressures or jerks. The spine protects your spinal cord, which connects your brain to other body parts (*A Patient's Guide to Anatomy and Function*, n.d.). It's important to take good care of your spine by being responsive to the signals it sends you such as pain or discomfort, and don't hesitate to consult your healthcare provider when needed.

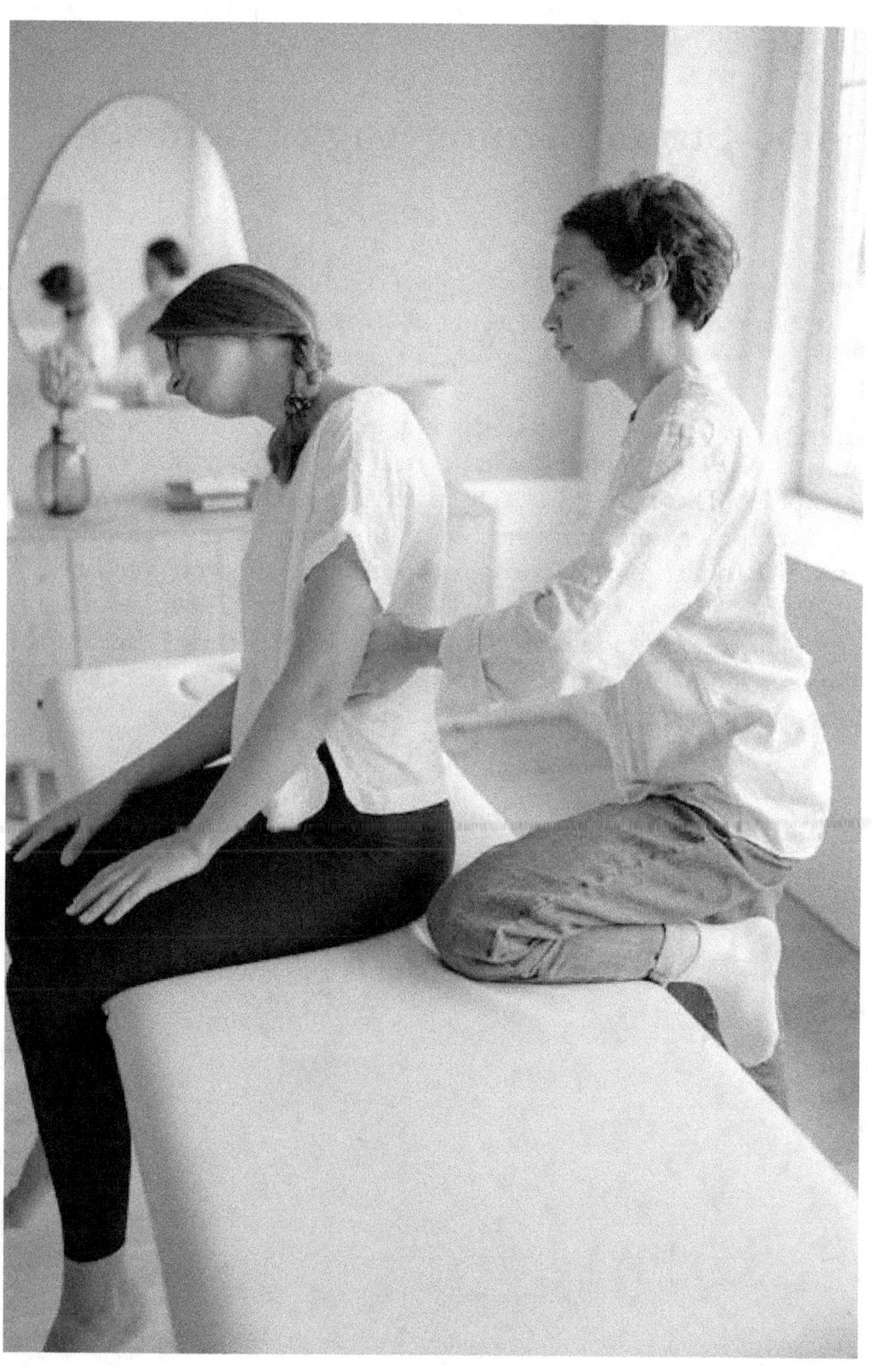

Focusing on Spine Health

A healthy spine is important for your overall functional fitness. Here are some tips to improve your spinal health (Tannous, 2021):

- Maintain good posture when you're sitting, standing, or walking.

- Exercise regularly and focus on strengthening your core.

- Use efficiently designed furniture and tools that support spinal health.

- Lift heavy objects correctly, bending at the knees and keeping the back straight.

- Avoid sitting or standing in one position for long periods.

- Use a good quality mattress and pillows.

- Practice stress management techniques to reduce tension in the back muscles.

- Stay hydrated to keep spinal discs properly hydrated and flexible.

- Avoid smoking as it can impair blood flow to the spine.

- Schedule regular checkups with a healthcare professional for preventive care and early detection of spinal issues.

Since your spine supports the body's structure and mobility, a weak spine can result in back pain, poor posture, or even spinal misalignment and affect your daily living. Bad posture can affect your spinal health negatively.

Learning and regularly practicing spine-stabilizing and core-strengthening exercises can help you prevent back discomfort, improve posture, and maintain spinal health.

A strong core helps keep your back straight and balanced, preventing problems like slouching or back pain. It's like having a strong foundation that supports your spine and keeps it in the right position, making it less likely for you to hurt your spine. Major core muscles include the rectus abdominis, the obliques, the transverse abdominis, the erector spinae, and pelvic floor muscles. These muscles work together to provide stability, support, and control for movements involving the spine, pelvis, and hips. Strengthening the core muscles is essential for overall stability, balance, and posture (American Council on Exercise, 2013).

Stabilizing the Spine, Improving Posture, and Relieving Back Pain Through Exercise

A strong core helps distribute your body weight evenly, reducing strain on the lower back and guarding against lower back pain that can be common among the elderly. Regular core workouts also strengthen the muscles surrounding the spine. These exercises typically involve movements that require stabilization of the spine and pelvis, such as planks, crunches, bridges, and rotational exercises. As these muscles are repeatedly engaged and challenged during workouts, they adapt by becoming stronger and more resilient, providing greater support and stability to the spine.

Let's look at a few simple exercises that you can include in your daily exercise regimen.

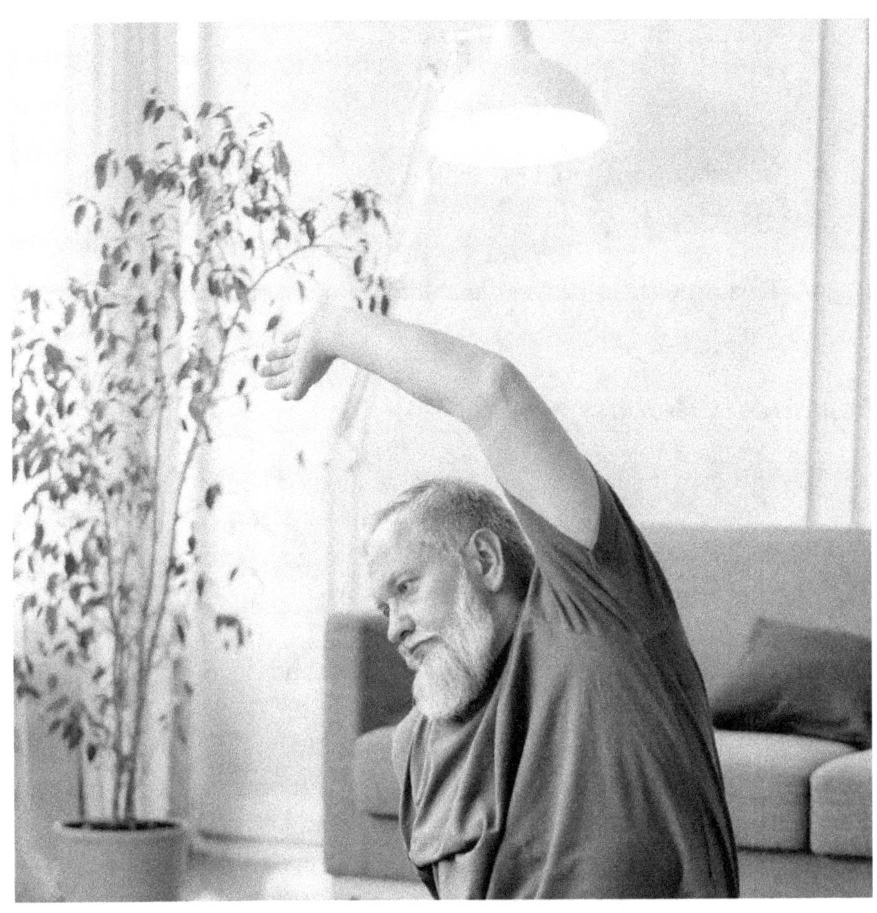

Seated Forward Folds

1. Sit on your chair with your spine straight and legs extended with your feet flexed up and resting on your heels.

2. Breathe deeply and bend forward to touch your toes.

3. Do not overexert to reach the toes; you can touch anywhere on your shins that you can reach comfortably while still getting a good stretch.

4. Hold the stretch for a moment before sitting back up.

5.   Repeat the exercise 3–5 times.

Benefits:

- Seated forward folds stretch the hamstrings, lower back, and spine.

- This exercise improves flexibility in the hamstrings and spine.

Seated Side Bends

1.   Sit on a chair with your legs extended or bent at the knees.

2.   Raise your right hand and hold the edge of the chair with your left hand.

3.   Reach your right arm over your head and bend to the left.

4.   Sit back up straight and switch hands, holding the chair with your right hand and stretching your left arm over your head to the right.

5.   Repeat the exercise 5–10 times.

Benefits:

- Side bends tone the muscles along the sides of the torso, which help stabilize and support the spine.

Seated Spinal Twists

1.   Sit on the chair slightly away from the backrest.

2.   Inhale and twist to the right. You can grab the backrest with your hands if needed.

3. Hold for a moment before returning to center.

4. Inhale and twist to the left.

5. Repeat the exercise 5 times on each side.

Benefits:

- This exercise can relieve back pain by toning and lengthening the spinal muscles.

- Spinal twists stimulate digestion.

- This exercise reduces tension in the back and hips.

Seated Cobra Pose

1. Sit comfortably on your chair with your spine in an upright position.

2. Exhale as you engage your core muscles and slowly begin to lift your chest and arch your back, keeping your shoulders relaxed.

3. Keep your neck aligned with your spine and avoid straining or tilting your head too far back.

4. Hold this position for 5–10 counts.

5. To release, slowly lower your chest back down and straighten your spine.

Benefits:

- Seated cobra pose helps strengthen the muscles along the spine, particularly the erector spinae, which run along the length of the spine and provide support and stability.

- It helps align your spine.

- When practiced with proper alignment, the cobra pose can help stretch and strengthen the muscles along the spine, which may alleviate tension and discomfort in the back.

Seated Pelvic Tilts

1. Sit up straight on your chair.

2. Keep your hands on your thighs or beside your hips for support.

3. Pull your navel toward the spine while inhaling.

4. Exhale and move your lower back slightly forward by gently tipping your hips forward to engage your pelvic muscles. Imagine you're making a very small arch with your lower back as if you're trying to slide your belt buckle forward. Use your abdominal muscles to do this, not your back muscles, as you need to feel a slight squeeze in your belly.

5. Hold for a few seconds, keeping your core engaged, then inhale and return to the starting position.

6. Repeat the movement 4-6 times.

Benefits:

- Seated pelvic tilts make your core muscles stronger.

- They improve pelvic mobility and flexibility.

- These exercises can ease lower back discomfort.

- Regular practice can enhance your posture and spinal alignment.

Shoulder Blade Squeeze

1.   Sit up with your back straight on your chair.

2.   Squeeze your shoulder blades together behind you while keeping your chest open.

3.   Hold for a moment then return to the initial position.

4.   Repeat the exercise 4–6 times.

Benefits:

- This exercise targets the muscles between the shoulder blades, helping to improve posture.

- The shoulder blade squeeze relaxes your neck and upper back.

- It supports spinal health.

Reverse Prayer Pose

1.   Sit up straight on your chair with your shoulders relaxed.

2.   Inhale, bringing your hands behind your back and entwining the tips of your fingers.

3.   Exhale and lower your chin toward your chest, keeping the back of your neck long.

4.   Maintain this pose for a count of 5–10 and notice your chest and shoulders expanding.

5.   To release, unwind your fingers and slowly lower your arms back down to your sides.

6. Take a moment to notice any sensations in your body before returning to a comfortable seated position.

Benefits:

- This exercise improves spinal strength and flexibility.

- Reverse prayer pose enhances core strength and posture.

Spinal twists, forward folds, and side bends are yoga exercises that can also be found in Pilates and general fitness routines because they offer benefits such as improving spinal mobility, flexibility, and core strength.

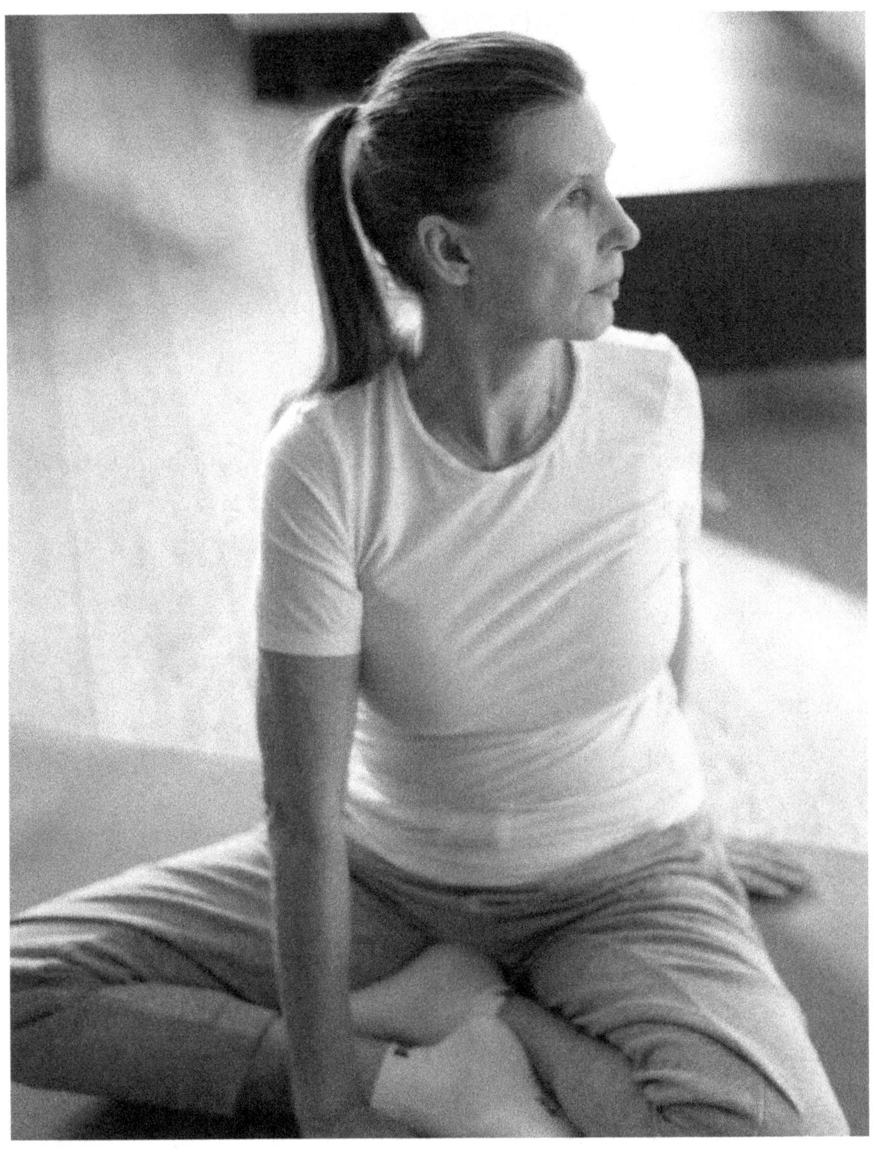

Lying Poses for Strengthening Your Spine

In addition to chair exercises, a few lying poses can help strengthen your spine. If you find it difficult to lie on a yoga mat or get up from it, you can perform lying poses in the comfort of your bed. Doing stretching exercises while lying on your bed awakens your body and mind, increasing your energy and alertness. Let's take a look at some lying exercises that can benefit your spine and your mind.

Knee-to-Chest Stretch

1. Lie on your back and pull your right knee toward your chest while keeping the left leg extended or bent, whichever is more comfortable for you.

2. Hold for a moment, feeling the stretch in your hamstring and hip, then straighten your right leg and repeat the stretch with your left leg.

3. Stretch each leg 3–5 times.

Benefits:

- This stretch tones the lower back and glutes.

- The knee-to-chest stretch enhances the strength and resilience of the spine.

- It enhances the range of motion of the hip flexor muscles.

Rotational Stretch

1. Lie on your back with your knees bent and feet resting flatly on the bed.

2. Stretch your arms out to each side at chest level and let them rest on the bed.

3.   Keep your knees together and slowly lower them to the right to rest on the bed while turning your head to look to your left. Remember to breathe.

4.   Maintain the position for 10 seconds.

5.   Return your knees to center, then repeat the motion by lowering your knees to the left and turning your head to the right. Don't forget to breathe!

6.   Hold for a count of 10.

Benefits:

- This stretch enhances the elasticity and agility of the muscles of your core.

- The rotational stretch provides relief from back discomfort.

Full Body Stretch

1.   Lie on your back with your legs extended and your arms stretched overhead.

2.   Point your toes and reach your fingers away from your body.

3.   Inhale deeply.

4.   Exhale slowly as you engage your core and gently press your lower back into the bed.

5.   Stretch your body as long as possible, keeping your hands overhead and feeling the lengthening of your body from fingertips to toes.

6. Maintain the stretch for 15–30 seconds while taking deep, steady breaths.

7. Release and repeat 2–3 times.

Benefits:

- This exercise is widely practiced by Pilates, yoga, strength training, and cardio practitioners alike as it lengthens and elongates the muscles, improving overall flexibility.

- The full body stretch boosts circulation and relaxes your muscles.

- It relieves muscle tension and tightness, particularly in the back, hamstrings, and shoulders, and improves posture.

- This exercise makes your joints agile and elastic.

- The full body stretch promotes relaxation and a sense of well-being through deep breathing and mindful movement.

A strong and well-aligned spine is indeed a fundamental precursor to balance and stability. Thus, after nurturing your spinal health, empower yourself further with exercises that improve your balance and stability by flexing and stabilizing the muscles in your legs.

Chapter 6:

Building Balance and Stability With Seated Poses

Balance is not something you find, it's something you create. –Jana Kingsford

As you move forward in your life's journey, you may face challenges in keeping your muscles strong enough to manage your weight and maintain your balance and stability. Both physical and mental balance play a role in helping you lead an independent life. In this chapter, we'll explore how you can improve your mental and physical equilibrium with chair workouts that help improve your balance and stability, making every sit an opportunity for strength and poise.

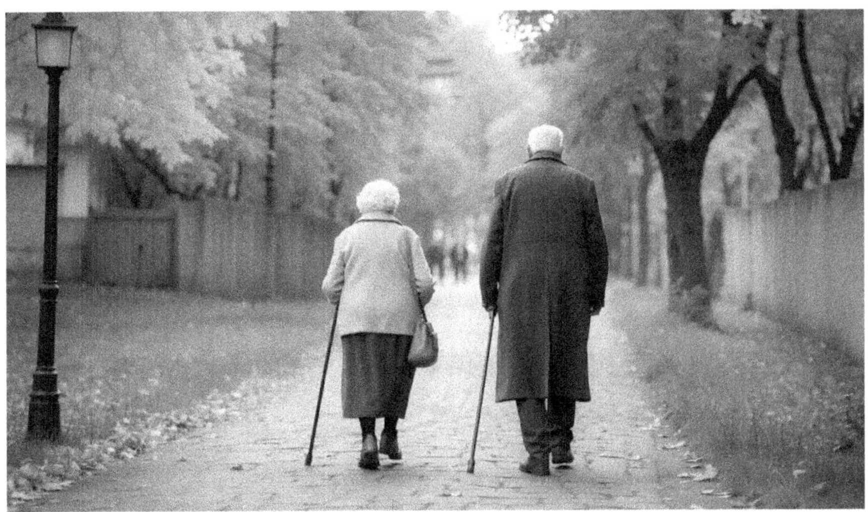

The Benefits of Balance and Stability for Seniors

Enhancing balance and stability as you age is essential for:

- **Improving mobility and independence:** Better balance enables you to maintain greater mobility and independence in your daily activities.

- **Reducing the risk of falls:** Improving your balance and stability through targeted exercises can significantly decrease the likelihood of falls, thereby preventing potentially serious injuries.

- **Increasing confidence:** Good control over your body leads to improved balance, which allows you to move around with more confidence and ease both indoors and outdoors.

- **Improving your quality of life:** As you feel more secure in your ability to maintain your balance, you can engage in more physical and social activities. This contributes to a better quality of life and overall well-being.

Some Points to Ponder

Here are a few things to keep in mind while exercising:

- Include balance and stability exercises in your regular routines to achieve incremental progress over time.

- Begin with basic exercises and progressively raise the challenge as your balance and stability improve.

- Practice balance exercises in a safe area and use a strong chair or support if necessary to avoid falls or injuries.

- Maintain appropriate posture and alignment to maximize the benefits to your stability and balance.

Improving Balance and Stability With Chair Routines

In this section, we'll discuss some exercises that focus on strengthening your leg muscles and developing good control over your body through proprioception to help you maintain or develop good balance.

Seated Leg Extensions

This exercise is also called seated leg lifts or seated leg raises.

1. Sit comfortably on your chair slightly away from the backrest.

2. Extend your right leg straight out in front of you with your left foot resting flat on the floor.

3. Hold your leg in the extended position for 5–10 counts, then bring it down.

4. Repeat the exercise with your left leg extended and right foot on the floor.

5. Do 5–10 extensions with each leg.

Benefits:

- This exercise works the quadricep muscles in the front of the thighs as well as the abdominal muscles and hip flexors.

- Leg extensions boost strength and stability in the leg muscles.

Tip:

- Pull your toes toward yourself while extending your legs to engage the calf muscles and get a better stretch.

Seated Tree Pose

1. Sit up straight on your chair before you begin this exercise.

2. Lift your right foot off the floor and place its sole on your left calf or inner thigh. Be sure not to place it on your knee joint.

3. Keep your hands on your thighs or bring them together in front of your chest in a prayer position (*Anjali* mudra, explained in detail in Chapter 9) for balance.

4. Engage your core muscles and lengthen through your spine, finding a steady focal point to help you balance.

5. Breathe deeply and hold the position for several breaths, maintaining balance and stability.

6. Lower your right foot down and repeat the exercise with your left foot.

7. Do the stretch 3–5 times with each leg.

Benefits:

- Seated tree pose helps improve balance, focus, and concentration.

- It works your hips, inner thighs, and groin muscles.

Chair Pose With Support

1. Place your chair facing a wall and sit with your back straight and feet flat on the floor.

2. Stand up and place your hands on the wall for support.

3. Inhale deeply, making sure your back is straight.

4. Exhale as you bend your knees and lower your hips as if sitting back in the chair but don't sit down.

5. After holding the chair pose for a few counts, push through your heels to stand back up.

6. Remember to keep breathing deeply throughout the exercise.

7. Repeat the exercise 4–5 times.

Seated Calf Raises

1. Sit on your chair with your knees bent.

2. Place a dumbbell on top of your thighs near your knees to add resistance if desired. You can make the exercise easier by not using the external weight.

3. Maintain a straight posture.

4. Inhale and raise your heels off the ground as high as is comfortable while contracting the calf muscles and pushing down through the toes and balls of your feet.

5. Hold the raised position for 5 counts.

6. Inhale and slowly lower your heels back down.

7. Perform 2–3 sets of seated calf raises. You may rest for a few seconds between sets.

8. As you get stronger, you can increase the number of sets or add or adjust the additional weight to provide more resistance.

Benefits:

- Calf raises engage the muscles of the calf and reduce strain on the lower back.

- They allow focused concentration on calf muscles.

- This exercise is suitable for injury rehabilitation and strengthening the calf muscles.

Advanced Calf Raises With a Chair

1. Stand tall facing your chair, holding the backrest for support.

2. Inhale and lift your heels off the ground as high as you can, pressing into the ground through your toes.

3. Maintain this position for a count of 5 while squeezing your calf muscles.

4. Slowly lower your heels back down to the floor and exhale, feeling a stretch in your calf muscles.

5. Aim for 2–3 sets of calf raises, resting for a few moments between sets.

6. Maintain proper form throughout the exercise and avoid any bouncing or jerking movements.

Benefits:

- Standing calf raises work both the big and small calf muscles.

- This exercise strengthens your calves, improving your ability to balance your weight.

- It creates a greater range of motion for your calves.

A Sequence to Improve Your Gait

As you advance in your chair yoga practice and feel your flexibility and balance improving, you can challenge yourself by:

- Doing more repetitions of the exercises included in your workouts.

- Trying more difficult poses.

- Increasing the duration of holding a pose.

- Performing simple standing poses with support.

Challenging yourself is important but not at the cost of your safety. Ensure safety by listening to your body's signals like pain, tiredness, or increased heart rate. Do not hesitate to rest or take a water break during your workout. Additionally, do not forget the golden rule of starting your session with at least 5–10 minutes of warming up and finishing it with a 5–10 minute cool-down session.

Let's now look at an exercise sequence that combines five exercises to be performed in succession to take your balance, stability, and gait to the next level and mitigate the risks of falls. You can use a wall, pillar, or your chair as a support while performing these standing exercises (Ennis, 2023):

One: Sit to Stand

1. Rest your palms on your thighs and feet flat on the floor as you sit comfortably in your chair.

2. Stand up from the chair, exhaling and pressing your palms into your thighs for assistance if needed.

3. Hold for a moment before sitting back down on the chair.

4. Repeat 2–3 times.

Two: Hip Abduction

1. Stand up straight with your hands on your waist to balance your weight.

2. Lift your right leg slightly off the ground and gently swing it from side to side slightly out in front of you.

3. Swing back and forth a few times before putting your right foot back down.

4. Repeat the swinging motion with your left leg.

5. Incorporate deep breathing with the exercise, inhaling as you lift your leg sideways (abduction) and exhaling as you bring your leg back to the starting position (adduction).

Three: Standing on Your Toes

1. Rest your hands on your waist as you stand up straight.

2. Take a step forward with your right foot.

3. Lift your heels to stand on your toes.

4. Hold for a moment, then step your right foot back.

5. Step forward with your left foot and repeat the exercise.

6. Relax your mind and body by breathing deeply throughout the exercise.

Four: Staggered Stance Position

1. Stand up straight with your feet about shoulder-width apart.

2. Extend your arms in front of you, joining your palms without bending your elbows.

3. Keeping your left arm pointing forward, rotate through your waist and torso to the right, bringing your right arm around with the rotation.

4. Hold for a moment then return to center.

5. Repeat the exercise by twisting to the left.

Five: Staggered Stance With a Yoga Strap

1. Stand up straight with your feet hip-width apart.

2. Stretch your arms out straight in front of you and hold a yoga strap tightly with both hands.

3. Twist your upper body to the right with your arms still straight out from your shoulders.

4. Hold the position for a moment, then come back to the starting position.

5. Twist your upper body to the left, arms still straight and holding the strap.

6. Hold for a moment, then return to center.

The exercises in this sequence increase in difficulty with each step. You can begin by performing the exercises individually and then add on the next steps based on your progress. Follow the full sequence only when you feel comfortable doing so.

Exploring Inner Equilibrium

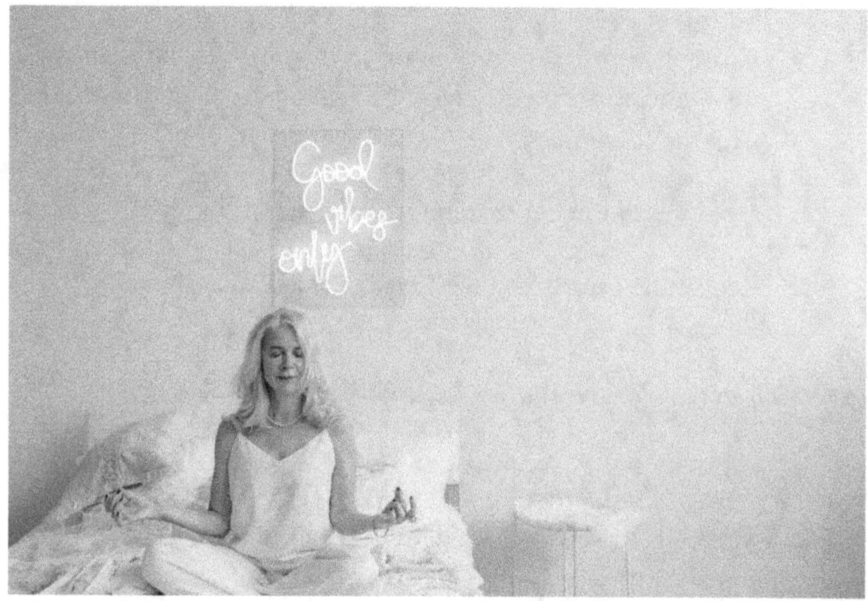

Cultivating mental and emotional stability complements physical balance. Mindfulness, meditation, and stress management can help enhance your inner equilibrium and overall well-being. By nurturing your inner equilibrium alongside your physical stability, you can achieve a harmonious balance that promotes health and vitality in your later years.

Mindfulness makes you more aware and enhances your sense of body position, or proprioception, by reducing stress and improving your mental focus and concentration. Here's how you can improve your inner equilibrium for better balance and stability:

- **Mind-body connection:** Explore the connection between mental focus, physical awareness, and balance to establish inner stability through mindfulness practices. By developing a deeper understanding of the relationship between your thoughts and actions or movements, you can pave the way for better balance and stability.

- **Seated meditation:** Seated meditation practice helps increase present-moment awareness, relax the mind, and improve attention, all of which can help with balance and stability.

- **Breathing techniques:** Apply breathing techniques like diaphragmatic breathing and alternate nostril breathing to induce relaxation, reduce tension, and improve balance.

We will discuss meditation and breathing techniques in more detail in Chapter 9.

Balance and stability are necessary because they promote general confidence, mobility, independence, and quality of life, and they can help you avoid falls. By strengthening your muscles through exercise, you can enhance your ability to maintain equilibrium and boost your confidence as you stand, walk, and engage in other physical functions, all of which reinforce the importance of having a strong core.

Your core consists of a complex network of muscles, including the rectus abdominis, internal and external obliques, transverse abdominis, erector spinae, and multifidus. These muscles work together to stabilize the spine, pelvis, and hips, providing a solid foundation for movement and supporting overall posture and balance. The core serves as the anchor from which power and stability radiate throughout the body. Strong core muscles facilitate dynamic movement and safeguard against injury. In the next chapter, we'll unleash the full potential of your core strength.

Chapter 7:

Core Strength and Control With Yoga and Pilates

The whole country, the whole world, should be doing my exercises. They'd be happier. –Joseph Pilates

As a child, Joseph Pilates, the inventor of the Pilates exercise discipline, had developed weak muscles from rickets. To make them stronger, he learned and practiced yoga, martial arts, Zen meditation, and some Greek and Roman exercises. This knowledge helped him develop a set of 50 exercises that enabled the muscles to work against one's body weight. During World War I, Joseph Pilates was detained in a British internment camp and helped his fellow internees and wounded soldiers by attaching springs under their beds to help them exercise their muscles. This innovative approach yielded positive results, and the doctors also noticed the speedy healing. Pilates's innovative approach soon became famous and eventually evolved into the discipline that is practiced worldwide today (Kloubec, 2011). Integrating gentle Pilates exercises with chair yoga can enhance body awareness, core strength, and overall flexibility and foster a greater sense of mindfulness and physical empowerment.

Sculpting a Strong Core

Core stability is essential for everyday activities like sitting, standing, and walking because it provides a solid foundation for movement and balance. Incorporating core-strengthening exercises into your workout routine can play a crucial role in supporting the spine, improving posture, and reducing the risk of strains and discomfort.

The core muscles consist of several groups of muscles, including the rectus abdominis, the obliques, the transverse abdominis, and the erector spinae. These muscles wrap around the torso, providing stability and support to the spine and pelvis by maintaining proper alignment and resisting excessive movement. Together, they enable the spine to function while also reducing pressure on the spine.

Pilates exercises are effective in sculpting a strong core and improving overall flexibility, posture, and muscular endurance. They are performed while sitting or lying on specialized equipment called reformers, or they can be done on a mat laid on the ground. Experts also recommend the chair variation of Pilates, especially for those who face mobility issues (SeniorShape Fitness, 2021).

Yoga often incorporates meditation, breath work, and spiritual elements alongside physical postures, while Pilates primarily focuses on physical conditioning and strengthening exercises without the spiritual aspects. However, Pilates practitioners do incorporate mindfulness exercises, which aim to improve concentration, control, centering, precision, breath, and flow.

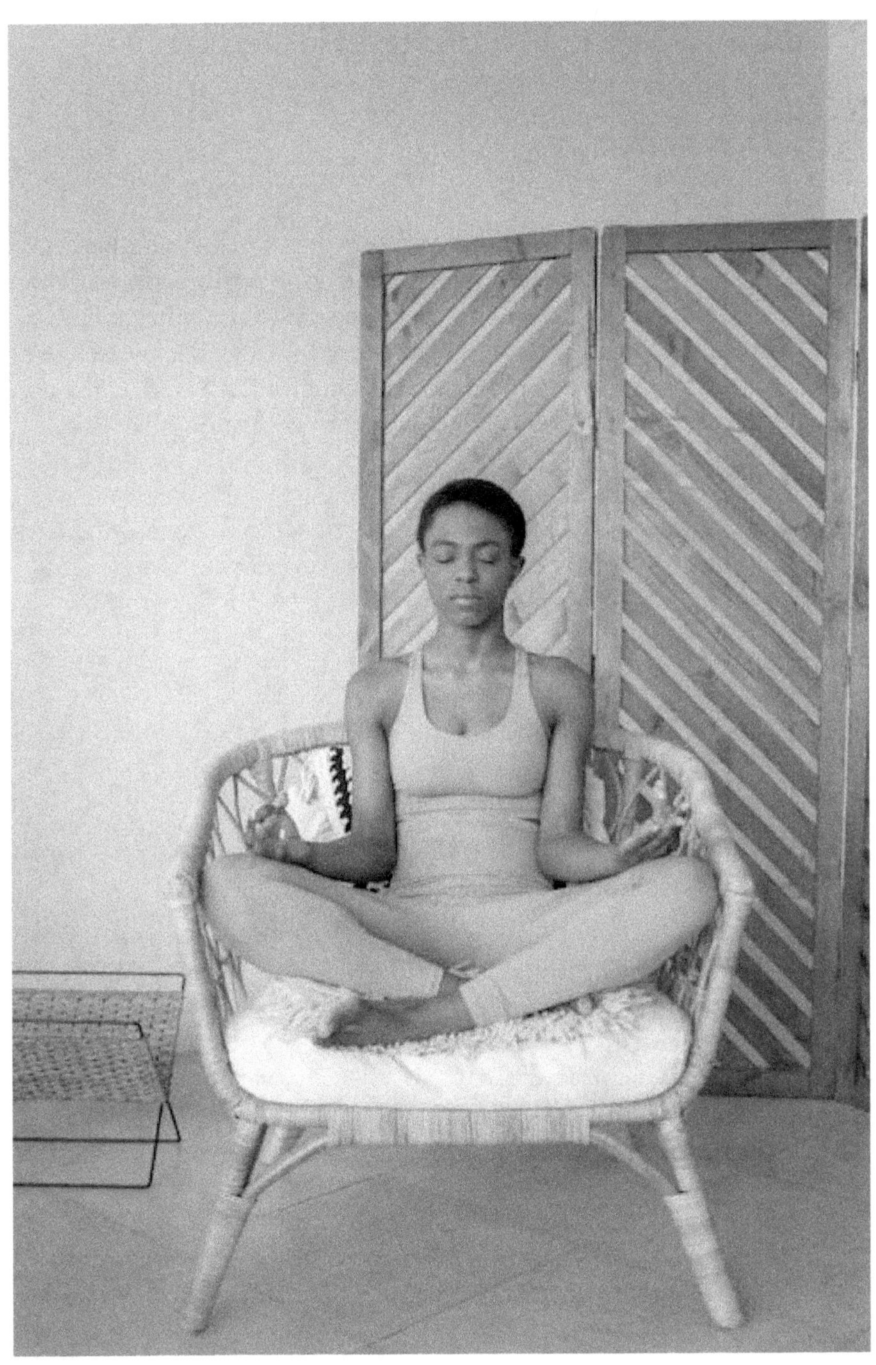

Pilates and Yoga: The Shared Core-Exercise Realm

Both yoga and Pilates involve stretching exercises that strengthen your core. Core strength is crucial for maintaining good posture and a healthy spine, which can help alleviate back pain and prevent injuries related to poor posture or improper spinal alignment. A few Pilates exercises overlap with yoga, including the plank, the hundred, the bridge, the cat-cow stretch, and the swan dive, each targeting core strength, flexibility, and improved posture.

In this section, we'll look at a few exercises that combine yoga and Pilates and are modified to be done while seated or lying down.

Reclining Hand-to-Big-Toe

1. Lie on your back and extend your right leg upward, touching the big toe with your hand.

2. Hold a yoga strap and wrap it around your foot's arch if you can't touch the toe while lying on your back.

3. Bend your leg to an angle of 90 degrees or less, based on your flexibility.

4. Hold for a count of 5–10.

5. Lower your right leg and repeat the exercise with your left leg.

Benefits:

- This pose is beneficial for stretching the hamstrings and relieving tension in the lower back, which can indirectly help with sciatica pain.

- The hand-to-big-toe exercise works the core muscles.

Tree Pose With a Chair as Support

As you progress in your seated practice, try this variation of the tree pose that uses the chair for support.

1.   Stand up straight facing your chair.

2.   Breathe deeply and engage your core muscles.

3.   Shift your weight slightly onto your left hip and put your right foot on the seat of the chair.

4.   Press your palms together in front of your chest.

5.   Focus on a point in front of you to help maintain balance. Keep your gaze soft and steady. Maintain a straight posture and keep your shoulders relaxed.

6.   Hold the position for a count of 5–10, breathing smoothly and deeply.

7.   Lower your right foot to the floor and repeat the exercise with your left foot on the chair.

Benefits:

- Tree pose is good for improving balance and stability.

- It stabilizes the core.

- This exercise enhances focus and reduces stress.

- It encourages good posture.

Cat-Cow Stretch on Chair

1. Sit on your chair with your feet on the ground, slightly apart, and your palms resting on your knees.

2. Inhale deeply as you arch your back, lifting your chest and chin upward.

3. Breathe out slowly as you round your back, bringing your chin to your chest and pulling your belly button toward your spine.

4. Repeat this movement, alternating between the arching and rounding of your spine.

5. Continue for 5–10 breaths, focusing on the gentle stretch in your spine and the opening of your chest.

6. Return to the original upright position and take a moment to notice how your body feels.

Benefits:

*   This exercise, utilized by yoga and Pilates practitioners, mobilizes the spine and increases shoulder, neck, and spinal flexibility.

Chair Plank: Beginner Level

1. Sit on the edge of your chair with your feet flat on the floor slightly more than hip-width apart.

2. Place your palms flat on the seat of the chair directly under your shoulders with your fingers pointing forward.

3. Move your torso forward without bending and press down with your hands and feet firmly, engaging your core muscles and lifting your glutes from the chair.

4. Avoid sagging or arching your back and keep your core engaged.

5. Hold the position for a count of 5–10, maintaining good form and breathing deeply.

6. To release, gently relax and lower your glutes back down to the chair.

7. Repeat the exercise 2–3 times.

Chair Plank: Advanced Level

1. Sit toward the edge of your chair with your feet flat on the floor, slightly wider than hip-width apart.

2. Put your hands on the edges of the chair seat, fingers facing forward.

3. Press your hands into the chair and press your feet into the ground.

4. Straighten your legs but keep your feet flat on the ground as you lift your hips off the chair, forming a straight line from your head to your heels.

5. Keep your shoulders down away from your ears and directly above your wrists and hold your body in a straight line without sagging or arching your back.

6. Hold the plank position for a count of 5–10, aiming to maintain good form and breathing throughout.

7. Lower your hips back down to the chair.

8. Repeat the exercise 3–5 times.

Benefits:

- The plank exercise boosts core strength.

- It enhances your stability and balance.

- This exercise strengthens the shoulders and arms.

- Chair planks provide a low-impact option for individuals with wrist or shoulder issues.

The Hundred: Chair Variation

1. Sit on the chair without resting your back on the backrest. Your feet should be flat on the floor.

2. Hold the sides of the chair for support.

3. Lift your feet and stretch your legs straight out in front of you.

4. Pump your arms back and forth by your sides as if you were running while breathing in for 5 counts and out for 5 counts, aiming for 100 pumps.

Benefits:

- This Pilates exercise improves stability and strength deep in your core muscles.

- It is good for your lung health and function.

- This exercise improves heart health and boosts energy levels.

- It helps maintain a good posture.

Bridge Pose on Bed

1. Lie on your bed on your back with your feet flat and knees bent.

2. Reach your hands to your ankles and hold them.

3. Press your feet into the bed, lifting your hips and forming a straight line from your shoulders to your knees.

4. Hold this pose for a count of 5–10 before lowering your hips back down.

Benefits:

- This yoga pose strengthens the back muscles, including the erector spinae and gluteus muscles.

- It opens the chest and shoulders.

- Bridge pose stretches the neck and spine, promoting better alignment and flexibility.

- It supports the lower back and improves stability by strengthening the core muscles.

- This exercise activates the thyroid gland, which is responsible for proper metabolism and energy balance in your body.

- It improves circulation and oxygenation, reducing fatigue and boosting energy.

Posterior Pelvic Tilt

1. Start by lying flat on your back on the bed with your knees bent and feet flat.

2. Keep your spine in a neutral position with a small natural curve in your lower back. Relax your pelvis and make sure it's in a comfortable position.

3. Gently engage your abdominal muscles by drawing your belly button toward your spine. This action helps stabilize your core and support your lower back.

4. Inhale to prepare, then exhale slowly as you tilt your pelvis backward, pressing your lower back into the bed. Imagine tucking your tailbone under and flattening your lower back against the bed.

5. Hold this position for a few seconds, keeping your abdominal muscles tense.

6. Release the tilt and return to the neutral position.

7. Repeat 4–6 times, focusing on controlled movements and maintaining proper form.

Benefits:

- The pelvic tilt is an important yoga movement as it engages many muscles like those of the spine, back, hamstrings, and abdominals.

- It improves strength in the core muscles.

- This exercise helps increase pelvic stability by strengthening the pelvic floor muscles.

More Pilates to Strengthen the Core and Improve Posture

In this section, we'll examine more chair-based Pilates exercises that you can incorporate into your chair exercise regimen.

Hip Circles: Beginner Level

1. Sit upright on your chair with your feet flat on the floor about hip-width apart.

2. Hold the sides of the chair for support.

3. Tighten your abs by pulling your belly button toward your spine.

4. Begin gently tilting your pelvis in a circular motion with your hips in one direction for 8–10 repetitions.

5. After completing the repetitions in one direction, reverse the movement and circle your hips in the opposite direction for the same number of repetitions.

6. Breathe steadily throughout the exercise, inhaling while starting the circular motion and exhaling as you come back to the original position.

7. Aim to feel a gentle stretch and greater mobility in your hip joints as you perform the circles.

Benefits:
- Seated hip circles help increase the range of motion in your hip joints, improving flexibility and mobility.

- Engaging your core muscles while performing seated hip circles helps stabilize your torso, strengthen your abdominal muscles, and improve posture.

- The rhythmic movement of the hips can improve blood circulation in the hip area and throughout the body.

- Seated hip circles can alleviate stiffness in the hips, especially after prolonged periods of sitting or inactivity.

Hip Circles: Advanced Level

1. Stand up with your feet about hip-width apart. You can face a wall for support if needed.

2. Draw your belly button in toward the spine.

3. Move your hips in a circular motion, keeping your feet planted.

4. Do 5–10 repetitions in one direction, then reverse the movement and circle your hips in the opposite direction for the same number of repetitions.

5. Aim to feel a gentle stretch and better mobility in your hip joints as you perform the circles.

Benefits:
- Standing hip circles engage the core muscles as well as the muscles around the hips and legs, challenging your balance and stability.

- The wider range of motion compared to seated hip circles allows for greater hip mobility and flexibility.

- This exercise works muscles throughout the lower body, including the hips, glutes, quadriceps, and hamstrings, helping to strengthen and tone these muscles.

The Swan Dive: Seated Version

1. Sit up straight on your chair with your hands holding the sides for support.

2. Take a deep breath and lengthen your spine.

3. Lean forward, exhaling slowly.

4. Extend your arms forward, allowing them to hover slightly above your knees.

5. Keep your gaze forward and your neck in line with your spine.

6. Hold the stretch for a moment.

7. Take a deep breath and sit back up.

8. Repeat the movement 4–6 times.

Benefits:

- The swan dive strengthens the muscles in the back.

- It helps improve spinal flexibility and mobility.

- This exercise stretches the chest and shoulders, which can offset the effects of hunching forward.

- The swan dive strengthens the core muscles.

Seated Pilates Teaser

1. Sit comfortably on the edge of your chair with your palms resting on your thighs.

2. Straighten your spine and pull your navel inward, inhaling deeply.

3. Exhale as you slowly begin rolling your back from bottom to top toward the backrest of the chair, one vertebra at a time, keeping your hands on your thighs.

4. Continue rolling until your upper back is resting against the back of the chair. Your spine should arch slightly from your lower back to where your upper back meets the chair's backrest.

5. Inhale at the bottom position, keeping your core muscles tight.

6. Exhale as you reverse the movement, rolling your spine back up to the sitting position, stacking each vertebra one on top of the other.

7. Repeat the exercise 3–5 times.

Benefits:

- The Pilates teaser strengthens your abs and hips.

- It increases mobility and flexibility in your lower back.

- This exercise engages and strengthens the pelvic floor muscles.

Sitting Roll-Ups

1. Sit on your chair with your legs straight out in front of you and
    your feet flexed.

2. Tighten your core muscles and extend your spine.

3. Breathe in and stretch your arms up over your head.

4. Exhale and slowly roll your spine down, reaching your hands
    toward your feet.

5. Keep your spine rounded as you lower down one vertebra at a
    time.

6. Once your hands reach your feet or shins, hold and breathe.

7. Inhale, then gradually sit back upright, exhaling as you return
    to the starting position.

Benefits:

- Roll-ups engage the abs and the muscles along the spine.

- This exercise focuses on core strength and mobility of the spine.

Saw Exercise on Bed

1. Sit comfortably on the bed with your legs extended out in front
    of you.

2. Flex your feet and keep them slightly separated.

3. Stretch your arms out straight to each side.

4. Take a deep breath and extend your spine.

5. Breathe out gently while turning your upper body toward the right foot.

6. Try reaching past your right foot with your left hand.

7. Inhale and return to the original position.

8. Repeat on the other side, trying to reach past your left foot with your right hand.

9. Do 5–10 repetitions on each side with slow, controlled movements.

Benefits:

- The saw exercise improves core strength and spinal mobility.

- It enhances torso rotation, which can improve everyday movements and posture.

- This stretch reduces stress in the shoulders and upper back.

Side Leg Kicks

1. Lie on your right side with your head resting on your right arm and your left hand on the bed in front of you for support.

2. Bend your right leg slightly for stability and keep your left leg straight.

3. Inhale and lift your left leg directly up off your right leg. Keep your left knee straight while lifting.

4. Exhale as you lower your left leg back down, but don't let it touch your right leg.

5. Lift and lower your left leg 5–10 times.

6. Switch to lie on your left side and repeat the exercise with your right leg for the same number of repetitions.

Benefits:

- Side leg kicks promote stability in your hips.

- This exercise strengthens the muscles along the side of the body, which improves overall balance.

- It improves your body awareness.

- Side leg kicks improve leg strength and endurance.

- They can help alleviate hip pain and discomfort by strengthening the surrounding muscles.

Mindfulness During a Chair Pilates Session

Being mindful while exercising helps cultivate a deeper connection between your mind and body. Here are some ways you can engage in intentional movement and breath awareness while performing chair Pilates for a holistic approach to fitness and well-being:

- **Attentive movements and body awareness:** Giving your full concentration to your Pilates practice is essential, so focus on breath control, precision of movement, and posture to maximize the benefits of your workout.

- **Incorporate Pilates breathing:** Deep breathing the Pilates way helps with core engagement, relaxation, and focus. In Pilates, the typical breathing pattern involves inhaling through your nose and exhaling through your mouth. Expand your ribcage laterally and into your back as you inhale, creating space for the breath to fill your lungs fully. As you exhale, draw your navel gently toward your spine to engage the deep abdominal muscles, helping to stabilize the core and support the spine (Manheim, 2023).

- **Visualize while performing Pilates:** During chair Pilates routines, some experts suggest incorporating visualization techniques such as your lungs being pumped up while breathing deeply or envisioning tension leaving your body with each exhale. This can help foster a stronger mind-body connection and enhance the effectiveness of the exercise (Futurefit, n.d.).

What Is Sciatica?

The sciatic nerve starts in the lower back, or lumbar spine, and extends through the buttocks down the back of each leg. Sciatica refers to pain that can occur along the path of the sciatic nerve in people of all ages, not just seniors. However, certain factors associated with aging like degenerative changes, muscular weakness, lifestyle changes, and bone spurs can increase the likelihood of developing sciatica in older adults. The most common cause of sciatica pain is a herniated disc, which means there is an overgrowth of the spine in the lumbar region (Mayo Clinic Staff, 2024).

Preventing sciatica in seniors involves a combination of maintaining spinal health, promoting proper posture, and addressing lifestyle factors that can contribute to nerve compression or irritation. Here are some preventive measures seniors can take (Mayo Clinic Staff, 2024):

- **Maintain a healthy weight:** Having too much body weight can put pressure on the spine, making it more likely to compress nerves. To help prevent this and lower the chance of sciatica, maintain a healthy weight by eating well and exercising regularly.

- **Avoid prolonged sitting:** Limit prolonged sitting or sedentary activities as these can contribute to muscle stiffness and decreased circulation, increasing the risk of sciatic nerve irritation. Take breaks to stand, stretch, and move around regularly throughout the day.

- **Exercise regularly:** Engage in low-impact exercises that promote flexibility, strength, and stability in the spine and surrounding muscles. Gentle exercises like yoga can help keep the spine mobile and reduce the risk of nerve compression. Strengthening the core muscles, including the abdominals and lower back muscles, can provide support to the spine and help maintain proper alignment, reducing the risk of sciatica. Activities like planks, bridges, and pelvic tilts can help.

- **Have good posture:** Maintain proper posture while sitting, standing, and walking to reduce stress on the spine and surrounding structures. Use ergonomic chairs and supportive cushions to maintain spinal alignment, especially when sitting for long periods.

- **Practice proper body mechanics:** Ensure proper body mechanics when doing activities such as lifting heavy objects or bending forward. Use your legs rather than your back to lift objects, and avoid twisting motions that can strain the spine and exacerbate sciatic nerve symptoms.

- **Drink plenty of water:** Drinking enough water helps your muscles stay hydrated and retain their elasticity. Dehydration can lead to decreased spinal disc height and an increased risk of disc herniation, which can contribute to sciatica.

- **Get regular checkups:** Schedule regular checkups with a healthcare provider to monitor spinal health and address any underlying conditions that may contribute to sciatica, such as arthritis or spinal stenosis, which is a medical condition characterized by the narrowing of the spinal canal.

- **Quit smoking:** Smoking can impair blood flow to the spine and accelerate disc degeneration, increasing the risk of sciatica. Quitting smoking can improve spinal health and reduce the likelihood of nerve compression.

Core strengthening exercises like cat-cow stretch, chair planks, and posterior pelvic tilts can be effective in preventing sciatica.

Advice for Progress and Safety

A good exercise regimen is one that challenges you without causing pain or discomfort. It prioritizes safety and proper form to prevent injuries while also promoting gradual progress and improvement. Here are some tips to ensure a sustainable and enjoyable core fitness journey with yoga and Pilates:

- Begin with basic movements and gradually increase the intensity and complexity of your chair Pilates practice as you gain strength and control.

- Listen to your body and alter activities to accommodate any discomfort or limits.

- If you have a pre-existing illness or concern, contact your physician before beginning any new fitness program, including Pilates.

Strengthening your core muscles is indeed essential for maintaining your functional fitness, and ensuring joint health is equally important for overall mobility and function. In the next chapter, you'll learn exercises to help your joints remain healthy and active.

Chapter 8:

Keeping Your Joints Happy With Chair Yoga

Life continuously shoots arrows at you; to survive, be flexible and be on the move because rigid and fixed targets are the easiest targets. –Mehmet Murat ildan

Gently nurturing your joints with movements and exercises designed to promote joint health can be the key to maintaining flexibility and freedom from discomfort, allowing you to fully enjoy your daily activities. Regular exercise not only strengthens the muscles that support your joints but also enhances stability and range of motion, reducing the risk of stiffness, swelling, and injury during both exercise and everyday tasks.

Consider this: Just like certain parts of your home need regular upkeep to function smoothly, your body's semi-movable and movable joints— like those in your knees and shoulders—require consistent care to stay agile and pain-free as you age. Think of it as giving your joints a tune-up for the journey ahead, helping you steer clear of issues like arthritis or discomfort that can crop up over time. Taking care of your joints involves doing daily tasks on your own in addition to exercising.

Now, imagine having a handy guide to help you navigate the complexities of your body's movable joints. The following chart gives you a better understanding of how your body moves and functions so you can take charge of your joint health and enjoy the activities you love (*Joints*, n.d.):

Type of joint	Function	Location
Ball-and-socket joints	Allows for a wide range of motion, like reaching for items and lifting objects.	Hip joint: Helps with walking and climbing stairs Shoulder joint: Helps with reaching and lifting
Condyloid joints	Enables movements in various directions; helpful for tasks like typing, writing, and gripping tools.	Wrist joint
Hinge joints	Facilitates movement in one direction, aiding activities such as walking, climbing, lifting, and bending.	Knee joint: Helps with walking and climbing stairs Elbow joint: Helps with bending and lifting
Pivot joint	Allows for rotational movement like turning your head to look around.	Neck joint, specifically the first and second cervical vertebrae
Saddle joints	Permits multiple planes of motion, aiding tasks such as grasping, writing, and holding objects.	Thumb joint
Gliding joints	Allows bones to slide over each other, enabling activities such as walking and standing.	Wrist and ankle joints

Understanding these different joint types and their functions can empower you to better maintain mobility and independence as you navigate daily tasks and activities.

Now, let's see what your joints are made of (*Joints*, n.d.):

- **Nerves:** Nerves provide sensory feedback to the brain regarding joint position, movement, and pressure, contributing to proprioception and coordination of movement.

- **Cartilage:** This is a firm, flexible connective tissue that covers the ends of bones in joints, providing a smooth surface for movement and absorbing shock.

- **Ligaments:** Ligaments are fibrous tissue bands that connect bones to bones. They help avoid dislocation of the joints.

- **Tendons:** Tendons are bands of connective tissue that attach muscles to bones. They pull the muscles, allowing the bones to move at the joints.

Common Joint Issues

Let's look at some issues with joints that seniors may experience due to aging and leading a sedentary lifestyle:

- **Arthritis:** A prevalent joint condition with various forms, such as rheumatoid arthritis and osteoarthritis, arthritis causes inflammation, pain, and stiffness that can significantly impact mobility and quality of life.

- **Stiffness:** Often a symptom of joint problems like arthritis, stiffness can restrict movement and affect daily activities, leading to discomfort and decreased flexibility if left unaddressed.

- **Inflammation:** A symptom of many joint health issues, inflammation can result in swelling, tenderness, and warmth around affected joints, contributing to pain and reduced function.

- **Sprains:** Though often associated with ligament injuries rather than chronic conditions like arthritis, sprains are also common joint issues. They can occur due to sudden twists, falls, or impacts that stretch or tear ligaments. This can lead to pain, swelling, bruising, and reduced range of motion. While sprains typically heal with rest and proper care, severe cases may require medical intervention to prevent long-term joint instability or weakness.

Joint-Friendly Exercises

The more you exercise your joints, the better their flexibility and overall health will be. In this section, we'll talk about some exercises that can help keep your joints mobile, active, flexible, and strong and reduce the risk of sprains, injuries, and pain.

Ankle Rotations on Chair

1. Sit up straight on your chair with your feet flat on the floor.

2. Lift the toes of your right foot off the ground, keeping your heel firmly planted.

3. Rotate your foot clockwise 10–15 times, then rotate it counterclockwise for the same number of rotations.

4. Lower your toes back down and repeat the rotations with your left foot.

Benefits:

- This exercise strengthens and flexes the ankle joints.

- Ankle rotations can reduce pain and stiffness in and around the ankle joints.

Wrist Circles While Seated

1. Get ready by sitting upright with good posture on your chair.

2. Straighten and fully extend your arms out in front of you, palms facing the floor.

3. Make a fist with both hands, keeping your wrists straight.

4. Rotate your fists in a clockwise direction 10–15 times, then switch and rotate in a counterclockwise direction for the same number of rotations.

5. You can vary the size of the rotations based on your comfort and range of motion.

Benefits:

- Wrist circles flex and strengthen the wrist joints.

- This exercise strengthens the muscles around the wrists.

Leg Raises on Bed

1. Lie on your back on your bed.

2. Keep your left leg straight on the bed and lift your right leg, keeping it straight. Lift it as high as is comfortable for you, hold for a count of 5, then lower it back down slowly.

3. Repeat the exercise with your left leg.

4. Do 5–10 raises with each leg.

Benefits:

- Leg raises strengthen the muscles around the hips and knees.

Leg Swings

1. Sit up straight on the edge of your chair with your feet on the floor. You can hold the sides of the chair for support if needed.

2. Lift and straighten your right leg out in front of you while keeping your left foot flat on the floor.

3. Swing your right leg back and forth in a controlled motion from your hip joint.

4. Keep the knee of the swinging leg straight but not locked and breathe steadily throughout the movement.

5. Stretch your hamstrings and hip flexors while swinging your leg.

6. Do 10–15 repetitions then lower your leg and put your right foot back on the floor.

7. Repeat the exercise with your left leg for the same number of repetitions.

8. Manage the intensity by adjusting the speed and range of motion. Be responsive to your body and take breaks when needed.

Benefits:

- Leg swings improve flexibility and mobility in your hip flexors and hamstrings.

Knee Presses on Bed

1. Lie down on your back on your bed. Rest your feet flat on the bed with your knees bent and feet separated.

2. Keep your arms along your sides with your palms facing down.

3. Draw your belly button toward your spine to help stabilize your pelvis and lower back while performing the exercise.

4. Keep your feet a comfortable distance apart and let your knees touch or come close together. Your thighs should be relaxed in this starting position.

5. While maintaining contact between your knees, press them together as firmly as you can without straining. Focus on using the inner thigh muscles to perform this movement. Hold the press for 3–5 seconds, feeling the muscles working in your inner thighs.

6. Slowly release the pressure and allow your knees to return to the starting position with a gentle natural separation between them.

7. Relax and breathe before repeating the exercise.

8. Repeat the exercise 10–15 times, gradually increasing the number according to your progress.

Benefits:

- Knee presses are a simple yet effective way to strengthen the inner thigh muscles and improve hip stability.

- They can also be used as part of a rehabilitation program for knee or hip injuries.

Seated Wall Push-Ups

1. Place your chair facing a wall and sit upright on your chair.

2. Place your palms on the wall at shoulder level.

3. Bend your elbows slowly, easing your upper body closer to the wall.

4. Pause for a moment then push yourself back up to the starting position.

5. Repeat the exercise 5–10 times.

Benefits:

- Seated wall push-ups strengthen the chest, arms, and shoulders.

- This exercise can help improve your posture.

Seated Row With Resistance Band

1. Sit on a chair with your legs straight and feet resting on the ground.

2. Wrap a resistance band around the bottoms of your feet, holding its ends with your hands.

3.   Pull the band toward yourself with your elbows pointing out to each side, engaging your shoulder blades and bringing them together.

4.   Release slowly.

5.   Perform the exercise 3–5 times.

Benefits:

- The seated row exercise makes your upper back and shoulders stronger.

- It mimics the pulling motion commonly used in daily activities. By strengthening the muscles involved in these movements, this exercise can help improve overall functional strength, making everyday tasks easier and reducing the risk of injury.

Warrior II (Virabhadrasana II)

1.   Sit tall on your chair with your feet planted firmly on the ground, hip-width apart.

2.   Stretch your arms out to the sides, parallel to the ground with your palms facing down.

3.   Maintain an upright sitting posture.

4.   Turn your left foot so that your toes are pointing to the left. Make sure your left knee stays directly over your left ankle.

5.   Turn your torso to your left.

6.   Step your right foot back, pointing the toes toward your left foot.

7.   Gaze over your left fingertips.

8.   Hold the pose for several breaths, breathing steadily.

9.   To switch sides, bring your feet back to the starting position
     and repeat the steps in the opposite direction.

Benefits:

- Warrior II makes your legs, arms, and core stronger.

- It stretches the muscles of the hips, groin, and chest.

- This exercise improves balance, stability, and focus and
  promotes a sense of confidence and empowerment.

Downward-Facing Dog (Adho Mukha Svanasana) With Support

1.   Stand facing your chair with your hands resting on the back
     about shoulder-width apart. You may choose to put the front
     of the chair against a wall to keep it from moving during the
     exercise.

2.   Step back until your body forms an upside-down V.

3.   Keep your feet hip-width apart.

4.   Press your hands into the chair, lengthen your spine, and
     straighten your arms.

5.   Engage your core and gently press your heels into the floor.

6.   Hold the pose for 10–15 counts.

Benefits:

- Downward-facing dog using a chair stretches the shoulders, hamstrings, calves, and spine while strengthening the arms and legs.

- This exercise improves blood circulation and promotes relaxation in the neck and shoulder muscles.

- It is also good for managing and even preventing sciatica pain.

Triangle Pose (Trikonasana)

1. Sit comfortably on the edge of your chair.

2. Extend your right leg out to the side and place your right foot flat on the floor, toes pointing to the right.

3. Keep your left foot firmly on the ground. If it feels good, you can also move it slightly to the side.

4. Inhale and straighten your back.

5. As you exhale, lean your torso to the right, reaching your right hand toward the floor or seat of the chair.

6. Reach your left hand up toward the ceiling, creating a straight line from your left hand to your left shoulder.

7. Keep your neck in a neutral position or gently turn your gaze up toward your left hand.

8. Hold the pose for a count of 5–10.

9. To release, inhale and slowly come back to the starting position.

10. Repeat on the other side by switching the position of your legs and reaching your left hand toward the floor or chair seat and your right hand toward the ceiling.

Benefits:

- Triangle pose done while seated on a chair stretches the hips, hamstrings, groin, chest, and shoulders.

- It tones the leg and core muscles, improving balance and stability.

- This exercise improves digestion and blood circulation.

Inner Thigh Squeeze

1. Lie on your back on your bed.

2. Bend your knees and place your feet flat on the bed about hip-width apart.

3. Place and hold a cushion or rolled-up towel between your knees.

4. Focus on your breath and tighten your stomach muscles by gently pulling your belly button in toward your spine.

5. Inhale deeply and then slowly exhale as you engage the inner thigh muscles, squeezing the cushion or towel between your knees.

6. Hold for a count of 8–10 while breathing deeply and gently. Keep your pelvis steady and try not to arch your back.

7. Inhale as you release the squeeze and allow your knees to separate gently, taking the towel or cushion in your hands.

8. Keep your core engaged and rest for a moment between repetitions.

9. Perform 8–10 repetitions. You may increase the number of repetitions as you become more comfortable with the exercise.

Benefits:

- The inner thigh squeeze is a general strengthening exercise that targets the inner thigh muscles.

- This exercise can be incorporated into various types of fitness routines, including yoga, Pilates, or general strength training programs.

Tips to Maintain Joint Mobility and Minimize Stiffness

The more you care for your joints, the happier and more pain-free they are. In this section, we will learn about ways to maintain joint mobility and minimize stiffness.

Integrate Frequent Movement to Lead an Active Life

Follow an active daily routine to avoid stiffness and enhance joint lubrication. Staying active by doing things like household chores as much as possible is beneficial for joint health in seniors. It helps maintain joint flexibility, strengthens supporting muscles, and improves overall mobility. Engage in activities you enjoy and remember to choose activities that are suitable for your fitness level. Chair exercises are convenient, low-impact, and helpful for people with different fitness levels in improving mobility, strength, and balance, but doing daily chores and activities on your own is equally crucial.

Maintain Good Posture and Alignment

Be mindful of maintaining good posture and alignment while doing work or exercising to reduce joint strain and avoid spraining or overstretching tendons or ligaments. Keeping your back straight minimizes strain on your muscles and joints.

Incorporate a Warm-Up and Cool-Down Session

A warm-up at the beginning of your exercise session prepares your joints and muscles for the movements you're about to do and helps you avoid stiffness. It also prepares your mind to concentrate on the exercises. A cool-down at the end of your exercise session helps you relax your muscles and joints and brings your heart rate down gradually.

Get Adequate Rest for a Successful Fitness Journey

Taking short breaks while exercising or performing your daily tasks is essential to prevent overexertion of your joints. Adequate sleep is crucial for managing joint pain, muscular discomfort, and tiredness and contributes to better mobility and flexibility. Additionally, not getting enough sleep can disrupt the balance of appetite hormones, which can lead to overeating and weight gain.

Stay Hydrated and Eat a Balanced Diet to Help Manage Weight

Staying hydrated has so many benefits, but it also helps lubricate joints, which reduces friction and discomfort during physical activity, so it's important to drink 8–10 glasses of water daily. A balanced diet and healthy weight based on the BMI scale play important roles in supporting joint health and minimizing inflammation as well.

Joints like your knees, hips, and ankles have to bear your body weight, so carrying excess weight can cause stress on these joints, exacerbate conditions like osteoarthritis, and make movement more difficult. Focusing on a balanced diet that includes plenty of fruits, vegetables, lean protein, and whole grains while limiting foods high in sugar, saturated fats, and empty calories can help you maintain a healthy weight.

Foods like fatty fish, nuts, seeds, fruits, and vegetables reduce inflammation, so incorporate these foods into your diet as much as you can. Reduce your consumption of processed foods, sugary snacks, and foods high in trans fats, which can contribute to inflammation that can cause increased appetite, high blood pressure, poor gut health, heart ailments, and insulin resistance, which is the precursor to type 2 diabetes.

Do Joint Friendly Exercises and Adjustments

Low-intensity workouts are safe for seniors since they are easy on the joints and support general joint health. Modify your workouts to accommodate your individual needs by utilizing a chair or bed for support or limiting your range of motion to avoid discomfort.

Consult With a Healthcare Provider

Taking a doctor's or nutritionist's advice can provide personalized guidance on weight management through your diet. Maintaining a healthy weight helps ensure you are not straining your joints. Your healthcare provider can also recommend appropriate physical activities and exercises that support your joint health and overall well-being.

Use Props While Exercising

Using props during exercise can support muscle and joint health, especially for individuals with specific mobility concerns or joint issues.

Props can provide additional support, stability, and resistance, enabling individuals to perform exercises with proper form and reducing the risk of injury. Let's take a look at some of the props available for you to use during exercise.

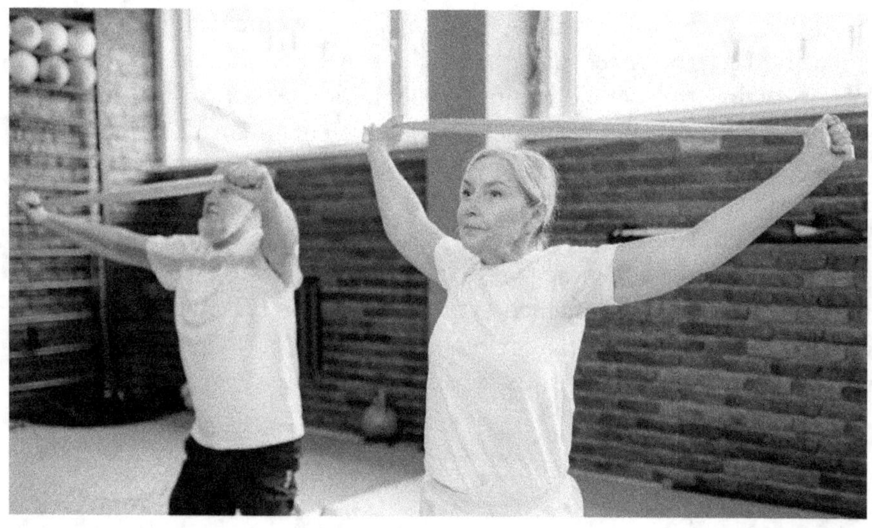

Resistance Bands and Yoga Straps

Resistance bands can help you strengthen the muscles around your joints by supporting and stabilizing them, which is especially helpful if you have joint issues. Unlike dumbbells, resistance bands provide you with different levels of resistance, making exercises gentler on joints. They're lightweight and can be used in a wide range of exercises, even while sitting or lying down.

Yoga Blocks

Using yoga blocks can assist you in achieving proper alignment during yoga poses, reducing strain on joints like the knees and wrists. Yoga blocks serve to minimize the space between the ground and your hands during poses where reaching the ground is challenging or impossible.

Stability Balls

These are versatile exercise accessories that can help you balance your weight better, make your core stronger, and improve joint health. Because they are made of either polyvinyl chloride (PVC) or rubber, they are anti-burst and inflatable. They offer enough support to help you maintain stability during exercises while also allowing for slight compression, which engages additional muscles to maintain balance. This dual purpose helps in strengthening the core muscles, improving posture, and enhancing overall stability. You can lean against a stability ball to engage your core muscles or use it to support your legs during leg extensions.

Cushions and Bolsters

These can be used to provide yourself added comfort while exercising, particularly in yoga and meditation, by providing support for various poses and promoting relaxation and proper alignment.

By incorporating props into your exercise routines, you can customize your workouts to your specific needs, minimize joint strain, and support your overall musculoskeletal health and function.

After ensuring your body is on the right track and functioning optimally, your mind also needs your attention. All aspects of your physical, mental, and emotional well-being are equally important and interdependent. In the next chapter, we'll delve into the realm of mindfulness, meditation, deep breathing, and restorative yoga to attain mental peace and relaxation.

Chapter 9:

Mindfulness and Relaxation With Yoga

Mindfulness means being awake. It means knowing what you are doing. –Jon Kabat-Zinn

Find peace and calm amid your hectic day with mindfulness and relaxation practices designed specifically for your sitting fitness practice. Before we proceed with the chapter, let's discuss how psychologists have defined mindfulness, meditation, and deep breathing so we can begin to gain an understanding of their role in relaxing your mind and body.

- **Mindfulness:** "It is a state of active, open attention to the present. This state is described as observing one's thoughts and feelings without judging them as good or bad" (*Mindfulness*, n.d.). Living mindfully involves cherishing the present moment and intentionally focusing on even the simplest daily tasks. It helps you to forget past traumatic or painful experiences and not worry about the future.

- **Meditation:** Meditation, called dhyana in Sanskrit, is a powerful tool that encompasses numerous practices that can help you achieve mindfulness, mental relaxation, calm, peace, and good health. It helps you have complete control of your mind and achieve calmness.

- **Deep breathing:** When you feel mentally or physically stressed, you automatically take shallow breaths, which sends signals to your brain to release stress hormones like cortisol and adrenaline. If you start breathing deeply when this happens, you are telling your brain that you are relaxed. Deep breathing activates the parasympathetic nervous system which then triggers the release of happy hormones like serotonin and endorphins, promoting a sense of calm and well-being. Endorphins are natural painkillers, and serotonin is a neurotransmitter associated with mood regulation, promoting happiness and well-being. Breathing mindfully also improves immunity.

Integrating Mindfulness and Relaxation Into Seated Exercises

Mindfulness can be a state of mind, a process, and a meditation technique. No matter how complex it is to achieve, it is essential for your overall well-being. Here is a list of important roles mindfulness can play in your life (Vago & Silbersweig, 2012):

- Mindfulness can lower your stress levels.

- It increases your awareness of the complexities of life and helps you develop self-awareness and self-acceptance.

- Mindfulness can help you develop mental clarity.

- Mindfulness leads to self-awareness, which can help you regulate your behavior.

- It encourages you to observe and regulate your emotions without judgment, allowing you to respond to them more constructively.

- Being mindful helps you develop empathy toward yourself and others.

As you can see, incorporating mindfulness into your life can have far-reaching benefits that contribute to your quality of life.

Meditation

Meditation helps cultivate attention and awareness and helps calm your state of mind, allowing you to observe your thoughts and emotions without judgment. It can help you focus on the present moment and do the task at hand with full concentration.

Although meditation is an age-old practice, understanding its effects on the human brain and body has been achieved through modern technology (*Meditation*, n.d.). Meditation is best done by sitting in a specific pose called an asana, forming a hand gesture called a mudra, and focusing your mind on your breath, a mantra, or a specific point of concentration to cultivate mindfulness and inner peace.

Asanas: Chair Variations

In this section, we'll go over some asanas that have been modified to be done while sitting on a stable chair.

Easy Pose (Sukhasana)

1. Sit up straight on your chair with your legs on the seat of the chair, crossed at the ankle. Rest your hands on your thighs.

2. Straighten your back and close your eyes.

3. Bring your awareness to your breath, breathing deeply and evenly.

4. Maintain this pose for at least 5–10 minutes, continuing to focus on your breath. If your mind wanders, gently bring it back to focus on your breathing.

5. When you're done, softly open your eyes, carefully uncross your legs, and take a moment to reflect on how you feel before carrying on with your day.

Benefits:

- Meditating in easy pose promotes a calm and relaxed state of mind.

- It can help improve your posture.

- This practice increases mindfulness and reduces mental and physical stress.

Butterfly Pose (Baddha Konasana)

1. Sit on your bed with your legs extended out in front of you.

2. Bend your knees and press the soles of your feet together. Let your knees fall open sideways.

3. Sit with your back straight. You can hold your feet or ankles during the stretch.

4. Gently press your knees down toward the bed, feeling the stretch in your inner thighs and groin.

5. Move your knees up and down in a gentle fluttering motion 5–8 times.

6. To release, relax your legs and extend them back out in front of you.

Benefits:

- This stretch targets the muscles inside the thighs and groin.

- The butterfly pose activates the organs in the abdomen.

- It enhances flexibility in the hip joints.

- This stretch can relieve minor back pain.

Mudras

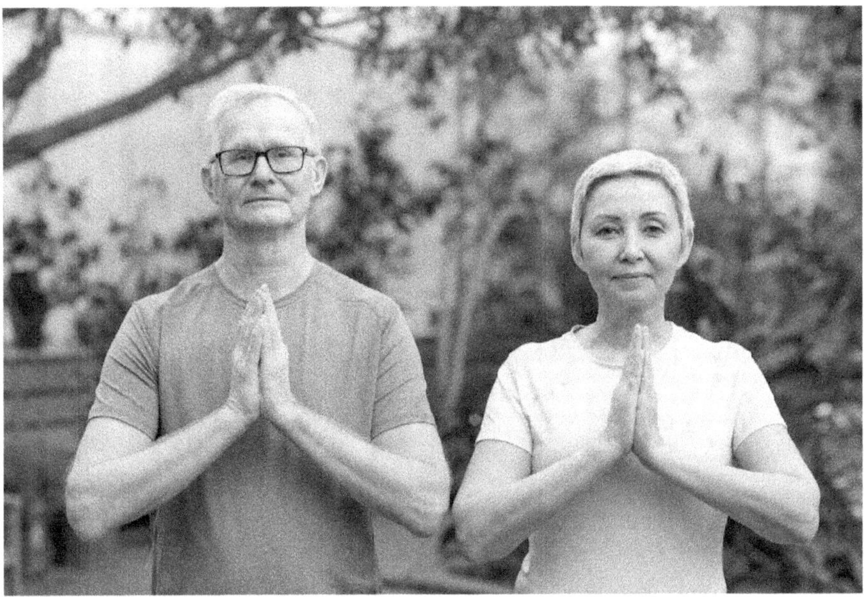

The hand gestures, or mudras, used in yoga and meditation practices help channel energy and promote various physical, mental, and spiritual benefits. In this section, we'll explore some common mudras.

Gyan Mudra (Gesture of Knowledge)

1. Sit in Sukhasana and keep your hands on your thighs with your palms facing up.

2. Touch the tips of your thumb and index finger together.

3. Extend the remaining fingers and keep them slightly apart.

Benefits:

- The Gyan mudra enhances concentration.

- This mudra can also improve memory and stimulate the brain.

Prana Mudra (Gesture of Life Force)

1. Assume the Sukhasana position.

2. Rest your hands on your thighs, palms facing up.

3. Touch the tips of your ring finger and little finger to the tip of your thumb while keeping the other two fingers extended.

Benefits:

- The prana mudra energizes your body.

- This hand gesture can help boost your immunity.

Dhyana Mudra (Gesture of Meditation)

1. Sit in Sukhasana and rest your palms on your feet.

2. Place the fingers of your right hand on top of the fingers of your left hand with your palms facing up.

3. Join your thumbs at the tips to form a triangle.

Benefits:

- The dhyana mudra calms the mind and enhances focus and concentration.

- This mudra can also promote inner peace.

Anjali Mudra (Gesture of Salutation)

1. Lightly press your palms together in front of your chest with your fingers pointing upward.

2. Allow your thumbs to lightly touch the chest.

Benefits:

- The Anjali mudra helps you maintain mental balance and calm.

- It can help you develop a sense of awareness of yourself and others.

Apana Mudra (Gesture of Digestion)

1. Gently press the tips of your middle and ring fingers against the tip of your thumb while keeping the other two fingers straight.

Benefits:

- This mudra can help improve digestion and remove toxins from the body.

Now that you know about mudras, you may incorporate them while meditating to help you focus better and experience the various mental and physical health benefits they offer.

Numerous brain scans show that when meditation is performed efficiently, the volume of gray matter increases. Gray matter is the part of the brain and spinal cord that is responsible for processing information, so an increase in the volume of gray matter indicates an improvement in the brain's functioning (Boccia et al., 2015). Meditation can be done in numerous ways, and in this section, you will learn about different ways to meditate and get a chance to practice them before choosing the one that seems most effective to you.

Prayer Meditation

1. Sit in Sukhasana and form Anjali mudra.

2. Shut your eyes and take deep breaths.

3. Say a prayer.

4. Open your eyes and get ready to practice other asanas.

Mindfulness Meditation

1. Sit or lie down comfortably on your bed then slowly close your eyes.

2. Take a couple of deep breaths, paying attention to how it feels as the breath flows in and out of your body.

3. Concentrate on your breath. Feel your chest rise and fall and the air passing through your nose.

4. If your mind starts to wander, gently guide your focus back to your breath.

5. Release any tension or discomfort you may be feeling with each exhale.

6. Acknowledge any emotions that arise, allowing yourself to experience them without getting caught up in thoughts or stories.

7. Expand your awareness to include sounds in the environment or sensations on your skin.

8. Remain present in the moment.

9. When you're ready to end your meditation, take a few deep breaths before opening your eyes.

10. Express gratitude for the time you've taken to practice mindfulness.

11. Return to your day, carrying the sense of presence and calm with you.

Affirmation Meditation

Affirmation meditation is a powerful practice that involves repeating positive statements, called affirmations, to cultivate a positive mindset, boost confidence, and promote well-being. Here are some simple steps to get started with affirmation meditation:

1. Choose a quiet and comfortable indoor or outdoor space where you won't be disturbed.

2. Sit on your chair in a comfortable position.

3. Start by breathing deeply and slowly. Inhale through your nose, filling your lungs, and exhale through your mouth, letting go of any tension.

4. Choose a few positive affirmations that feel right to you. Make sure they're in the present tense, positive, and personally meaningful. For example, "I am worthy of good health, independence, and happiness," "I trust in my abilities and decisions," or "I am grateful for all that I have."

5. Say your chosen affirmations aloud or silently. Focus on each affirmation one at a time, repeating it slowly and intentionally. Allow the words to sink in and evoke positive feelings within you.

6. Visualize yourself possessing the qualities or experiencing the situations described in each affirmation. Imagine yourself feeling confident, happy, and fulfilled as you affirm these positive statements.

7. Pay attention to how each affirmation makes you feel. Notice any shifts in your mood, energy, or mindset as you continue to repeat the affirmations.

8. To connect back to the real world, finish your meditation by gently wiggling your fingers and toes and opening your eyes.

Loving-Kindness Meditation

This kind of meditation involves cultivating positive feelings of love, compassion, and goodwill toward yourself and the people around you. Here are some simple instructions to get started with loving-kindness meditation (Kabat-Zinn, 2023):

1. Sit in a comfortable position on your chair with your back straight and hands resting lightly in your lap. You can also lie down on your bed during this meditation.

2. Close your eyes gently and take a few deep breaths to concentrate. Become aware of the sensations in your body and the rhythm of your breath.

3. Start by showing yourself love and kindness. Repeat these phrases silently or aloud: "May I be happy. May I be healthy. May I be safe."

4. Extend your love and kindness to others as well. You can start with someone you care deeply about, such as a close friend or family member. Visualize them sitting in front of you. Repeat the phrases for them and wish them well.

5. Continue to extend loving-kindness to other people in your life, such as acquaintances, coworkers, and even people you may have conflicts with. Gradually extend it to all beings, including animals.

6. Throughout the meditation, acknowledge without judgment any feelings that arise. If you encounter resistance or difficulty, gently return your focus to the phrases and the intention of cultivating loving-kindness.

7. Gradually finish your meditation practice. Take a few moments to reflect on the practice and nurture gratitude for the opportunity to connect with yourself and others in this way.

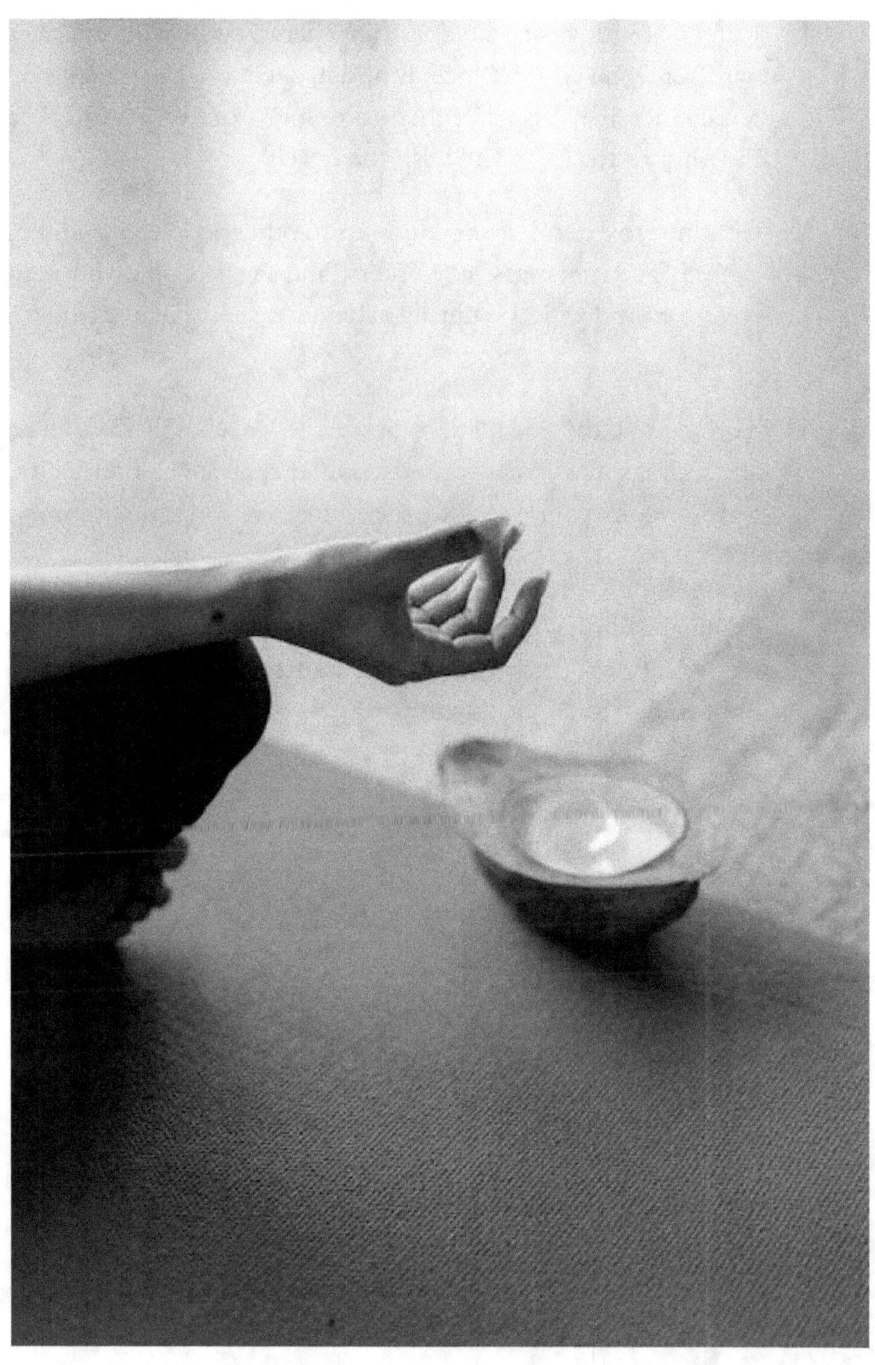

Body Scan Meditation

1. Find a quiet and comfortable place to sit on your chair with your feet flat on the floor, hands resting on your thighs, and your back straight but not rigid.

2. You can close your eyes or find a focal point to softly focus on.

3. Inhale deeply through your nose and exhale slowly through your mouth. Allow yourself to relax with each exhale.

4. Notice any sensations you feel in your toes, the arches of your feet, and your heels. Without judgment, simply observe any tingling, warmth, or pressure.

5. Slowly move your attention up through your body, focusing on each part individually. Notice the sensations in your ankles, calves, knees, thighs, and so on until you reach the top of your head.

6. As you scan each body part, gently release any tension you may feel in that area. If you notice any areas of discomfort or tightness, simply acknowledge them without judgment and breathe into those areas, allowing them to relax.

7. If your thoughts start to drift, gently bring your focus back to how your body feels, using your breath to help you stay centered.

8. Continue scanning your body from head to toe for a few minutes or for as long as feels comfortable for you.

9. At the end of your scan, slowly open your eyes and take a moment to notice how you feel before returning to your day (Raypole, 2022).

Visualization

Also known as guided imagery, this technique involves picturing tranquil and calming images to relieve tension and promote relaxation. Here is an example:

1. Imagine yourself sitting comfortably in a peaceful place, whether it's a cozy room or a serene natural setting.

2. Close your eyes and breathe in, imagining your body cells absorbing the fresh air.

3. As you exhale, visualize a warm, golden light floating down toward you, giving you a sense of calm and peace and washing away all your tension and worries.

4. As you continue to breathe deeply, visualize yourself surrounded by nature's beauty—perhaps you're sitting by a peaceful lake listening to the gentle sound of flowing water and the rustle of leaves or basking in the warm glow of the sun on a quiet beach.

5. With each inhale, draw in the serene energy of your surroundings.

6. With each exhale, release any lingering tension or negativity.

7. Try to take notice of every detail of the place and visualize yourself at peace.

8. Slowly open your eyes and carry out your daily tasks with renewed energy.

Grounding Exercises

Grounding exercises bring your attention to the present moment and connect you with your physical surroundings. These exercises are commonly used in mindfulness practices, therapy, and stress management techniques to promote relaxation and reduce anxiety. Here is an example of a grounding exercise:

1. Notice any five different colored things in your surroundings.

2. Pay attention to four different sounds, be it the sound of the breeze, the chirping of birds, the ticking of a clock, or distant music.

3. Smell any three things, ranging from the fragrance of nature, cooking smells in the house, or someone's perfume.

4. Touch any two differently textured objects.

5. Taste a citrus fruit.

This fun exercise helps you bring your awareness to the present moment by engaging all five senses.

Mantra Meditation

Mantra meditation is a technique in which the practitioner repeats a soothing phrase, affirmation, prayer, or word to relax their mind and build inner peace and tranquility. It reinforces the desired state of peace and calm. We'll look at a few examples of mantra meditation in this section.

Mantra: *Om Shanti* (May peace prevail in this world)

"Om" is believed to be the first sound of the Universe which encompasses all other sounds. It is considered sacred by many Asian religions, including Hinduism, Buddhism, and Jainism. Today, Om has transcended religions and cultures and is used by yoga practitioners as a form of spiritual and meditative practice. It is believed to have various benefits, including promoting relaxation, increasing concentration, improving heart and thyroid health, and creating a sense of unity with the universe (MasterClass, 2021). Some people break up the three sounds that make up Om (A-U-M) while chanting:

A long *A* sound

A long *O* (or *U*) sound

A long *M* sound

Chanting these sounds in a sequence invokes a sense of unity with the cosmos and a deeper connection to one's inner self or higher consciousness. It also improves the quality of your meditation session (MasterClass, 2021).

Breathing Practices for Stress Relief

Yoga establishes a connection between your mind, body, and soul, the three main aspects of your existence, through physical exercises called asanas and breathing exercises called pranayama. When performed regularly, these yogic exercises can offer relief from stress and anxiety by calming down the nervous system. They promote emotional regulation, improve sleep quality, and boost respiratory health.

Apart from incorporating gentle deep breathing while performing asanas, you can perform pranayama to take your deep breathing to the next level and derive even more health benefits from your workout. Pranayama exercises are commonly used in various relaxation techniques, meditation practices, and stress management exercises. In this section, we'll look at some common pranayama exercises you can perform to relax, achieve mindfulness, and release stress.

Diaphragmatic Breathing (Adhama Pranayama)

This breathing exercise is also known as belly breathing or abdominal breathing. It works your diaphragm, a large muscle located below the lungs that helps in breathing.

1. Get into a comfortable position, either sitting or lying down.

2. Relax your body as you close your eyes.

3. Put one hand on your chest and the other on your belly.

4. Inhale deeply through your nose, feeling your belly rise.

5. Exhale slowly through your mouth, feeling your belly retract.

6. Continue this breathing pattern for a few minutes, keeping your hands in place.

7. You can practice this breathing strategy each day to help manage stress and promote mindfulness.

Box Breathing (Sama Vritti Pranayama)

1. Sit with your back straight on your chair.

2. Close your eyes.

3. Inhale slowly through your nose as you count to 4.

4. Hold your breath for a count of 4.

5. Breathe out gently through your mouth for 4 counts.

6. Pause for another count of 4 before inhaling again to repeat the pattern.

7. Repeat this pattern 4–5 times.

8. Maintain a relaxed and steady pace throughout the practice.

9. Notice any sensations in your body and allow yourself to relax with each exhale.

10. Open your eyes gently when done.

Victorious Breath (Ujjayi Pranayama)

1. Sit comfortably on your chair with your back straight.

2. Take a deep breath in through your nose, gently tightening the muscles at the back of your throat to produce a soft hissing noise.

3. Exhale slowly through your nose, maintaining the same constriction in the throat.

4. Keep up this breathing rhythm for a few rounds, concentrating on the sound and feeling of each breath.

Frontal Brain Purification Breath (Kapalabhati Pranayama)

1. Sit on your chair in a comfortable position with your spine straight.

2. Breathe in deeply, then exhale forcefully through your nose by rapidly squeezing your abdominal muscles.

3. Let the next inhalation occur naturally without effort.

4. Repeat this pumping action for several rounds, gradually increasing the speed while maintaining the forceful exhalation.

Alternate Nostril Breathing (Nadi Shodhana Pranayama)

1. Sit up straight on your chair.

2. Use your right thumb to close your right nostril and breathe in deeply through your left nostril.

3. Release your thumb from the right nostril.

4. Use your right ring finger to close your left nostril and breathe out of the right nostril.

5. Breathe in through the right nostril, then close it with your right thumb and expel the air through the left nostril.

6. Repeat this process to complete one round.

7. Continue alternating nostrils for as many rounds as you'd like.

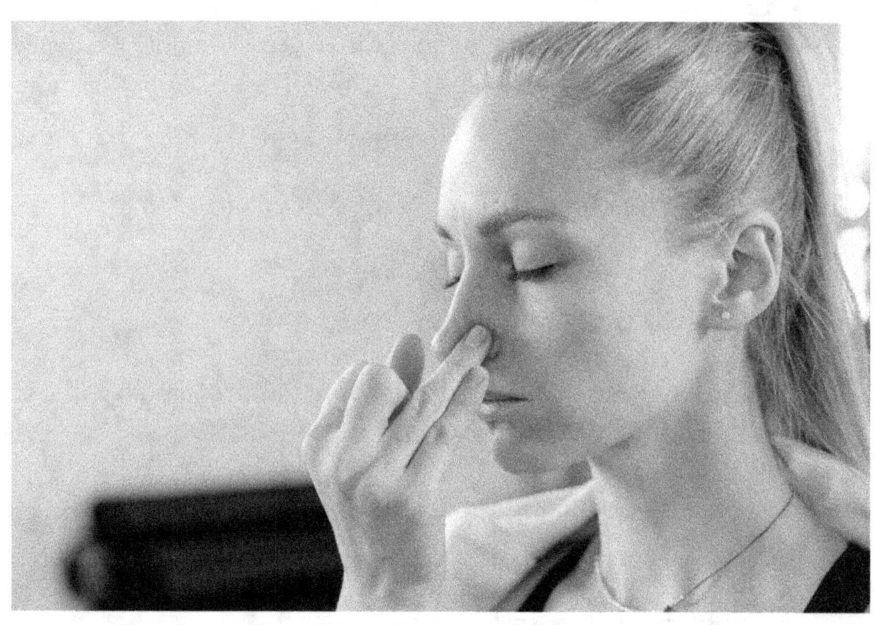

Bee Breath (Bhramari Pranayama)

1. Sit comfortably on your chair with your eyes closed.

2. Take a deep breath in through your nose.

3. Breathe out slowly while humming like a bee, keeping your mouth softly closed.

4. Repeat for several rounds, focusing on the vibration and calming effect of the sound.

Cooling Breath (Sitali Pranayama)

1. Sit comfortably on your chair with your back straight.

2. Roll your tongue to form a tube and purse your lips.

3. Inhale as if you're sipping from a straw through your rolled tongue and pursed lips.

4.   Close your mouth and breathe out gently through your nose.

5.   Repeat the breathing exercise 5–10 times, focusing on the cooling sensation of the breath (Arhanta Yoga, 2020).

How to Find Peace and Relaxation in Your Daily Practice

Practicing mindfulness and meditation supports your mental health and promotes relaxation. Here are some strategies you can adopt to make your journey more fulfilling:

- **Maintain a calm environment:** Minimize distractions and incorporate soothing elements like soft lighting, greenery, or gentle music.

- **Practice mindfulness regularly:** Set aside time to regularly practice mindfulness and relaxation and incorporate it into your daily routine for consistent stress reduction and well-being.

- **Pay attention to body sensations, breath, and your surroundings:** Concentrate on the sensations of movement and breath to deepen relaxation and awareness to maximize the effects of an exercise. Focus on your breath and allow it to deepen and guide your movements. With each inhale and exhale, bring awareness to the sensations in your body, fostering relaxation and mindfulness throughout the practice. Keep breathing even while holding a pose. By integrating these elements, you can develop concentration, establish a deeper mind-body connection, and experience greater benefits from your seated exercises.

- **Fix a spot:** Find a suitable place that is free of distractions in your home or workplace to perform your chair exercises to promote relaxation and mindfulness.

- **Strive to achieve mindfulness and relaxation daily:** Incorporating a variety of techniques into your chair yoga practice to help you reduce your stress levels and improve your overall well-being can give you faster results and help you live a more fulfilling life. Aim to include regular pranayama and meditation sessions during your exercise sessions or in between your daily tasks.

- **Approach your seated practice with self-compassion and acceptance:** Allow yourself to experience whatever thoughts or feelings come without judgment and practice showing yourself compassion. This gives you a positive outlook to embrace your strengths and shortcomings, enabling you to work toward personal growth.

Self-Care With Yoga

Some types of yoga can help you practice self-care to increase your well-being and boost your mood, energizing you to take on your day.

Restorative Yoga Poses

These gentle exercises are focused on relaxation and rejuvenation and involve using supportive props such as cushions, bolsters, yoga blocks, and yoga straps. Let's look at some of these restorative poses.

Corpse Pose (Shavasana)

1. Lie flat on your back in a comfortable position on your bed.

2. Extend your legs and keep your arms by your sides with your palms facing up.

3. Close your eyes and relax your entire body, allowing it to sink into the bed.

4. Take slow, deep breaths as you relax your mind and body.

5. Stay in this pose for several minutes, enjoying the sensation of relaxation.

Legs Up the Wall Pose (Viparita Karani)

1. Sit facing a wall.

2. Lie down on your back and place your legs on the wall. Don't bend at the knees.

3. Adjust your position so your buttocks are touching the wall or are as close to the wall as is comfortable.

4. Keep your arms at your sides with palms facing up or place them on your abdomen.

5. Close your eyes and relax, breathing deeply into your belly.

6. Hold this pose for several minutes to gently stretch your legs and promote relaxation.

Child's Pose (Balasana)

1. Kneel on the bed with your knees spread wide apart.

2.   Sit back on your heels and lower your torso forward, resting it on or between your thighs.

3.   Extend your arms forward, placing your palms flat on the bed.

4.   Rest your forehead on the bed or turn your head to one side for comfort.

5.   Breathe deeply and relax into the pose, feeling a gentle stretch in your back and hips.

6.   Hold this pose for several breaths or as long as is comfortable, focusing on deep relaxation.

Face Yoga

This type of yoga is a natural and holistic approach to rejuvenating your facial muscles and skin that promotes relaxation and enhances your facial appearance. Through a series of gentle exercises and techniques, face yoga aims to tone and lift the facial muscles, reduce tension, and stimulate circulation for a healthier, more radiant face.

Cheek Lifts

1.   Sit comfortably on your chair or bed with your back straight.

2.   Inhale deeply but gently, swelling your cheeks.

3.   Hold for a few seconds, then exhale slowly through your mouth, gently pressing your hands against your cheeks.

4.   Repeat several times to tone and lift the cheek muscles (Cronkleton, 2021).

Eye Circles

1. Sit comfortably on your chair with your back straight.

2. Roll your eyes gently clockwise 2–4 times then counterclockwise the same number of times.

3. Repeat several times to relax and rejuvenate the eye muscles, reducing tension and promoting circulation around the eyes (Cronkleton, 2021).

The Role of Community in Maintaining Your Health

Numerous studies have shown that spending time with a group of friends or family members works wonders in maintaining your health and well-being (Tiernan et al., 2013). Whether you engage in a big community or a small group of friends, you get ample opportunities to share opinions, release stress, and learn new things from others. Exercising in a group or with family members not only makes it more fun but enables you to learn the exercises faster. You can discuss your problems, find solutions, and devise ways to make them more enjoyable and result-oriented. Joining face-to-face yoga or Pilates classes or online classes can add more meaning to your exercise regimen. So go ahead and talk to your friends, neighbors, or family and enjoy a group workout!

A Yoga Sequence for a Healthy and Happy Mind

Whether you experience mental or physical stress, anxiety, or sadness, try this exercise sequence in the comfort of your home or in between tasks at work. You can do it either alone or with a group (Yoga Vista [aka YogaJP], 2013):

1. Sit upright on your chair with your feet hip-width apart and resting flat on the ground.

2. Breathe deeply throughout the exercise.

3. Say a silent prayer.

4. Rub your palms until they get warm.

5. Place your palms gently on your closed eyes and then massage your whole face.

6. Wrap your arms around your upper body.

7. Squeeze yourself gently at the shoulders. Release after 2–4 seconds.

8. Stretch your arms out in front and open and close your fingers.

9. Rotate your wrists.

10. Perform gentle spinal twists while seated in a flowing movement.

11. Engage in the seated side stretch exercise.

12. Perform leg extensions.

13. Bring your legs back to the original position and flex your feet so that your heels are resting on the ground and your toes are pointing up. Rotate your toes clockwise and counterclockwise.

14. Perform sitali pranayama.

15. Lie in corpse pose on your bed.

16. End the session with mantra meditation or loving-kindness meditation.

Now that you understand the importance of mindfulness in your daily life, you can incorporate deep breathing and meditation to attain peace and relaxation in your daily seated exercise. In addition to the physical benefits, yoga will be instrumental in bringing you mental tranquility, resulting in relaxation and quality sleep. Let us move on to the next chapter that guides you to find your fitness level, track your progress, and plan your customized exercise regimen based on your needs, mobility level, progress, and goals.

Chapter 10:

Building Your Personalized Chair

Fitness Routine

I've watched people who aged gracefully. And they all did some kind of exercise regularly. –Kay Willoughby

Being agile, active, and independent is the best way to enjoy your golden years, and designing a personalized chair workout plan that involves your favorite exercises can help you get there. Try to find a bright, well-ventilated, quiet corner in your home where you can place your chair and exercise daily. You may beautify the space with plants or play gentle music to keep yourself motivated.

Here are some more points to keep in mind while creating your chair fitness routine:

1. Evaluate your fitness needs and abilities.

2. Set your goals.

3. Create a personalized exercise plan.

4. Take care of your nutrition.

In this chapter, we'll delve into each of these steps so you have a clear understanding of how to create the chair fitness routine that will be most beneficial to you.

Evaluate Your Fitness Needs and Goals

Prioritize safety while exercising. Consider your fitness level, goals, and challenges before planning and beginning your exercise routine. This analysis will assist you in incorporating exercises that will help you achieve your fitness objectives without causing any negative side effects or discomfort. Measure your fitness level with the tips given in the chart below (Mayo Clinic Staff, 2023):

Factors to determine your fitness level	How the factors help you determine your fitness needs and goals
Your mobility level	Can you walk independently or with support? Your mobility indicates how well your joints move. Being aware of your mobility can be useful in choosing the right combination of exercises. If you have low mobility, you need to perform gentle exercises on a chair that work various muscle groups and joints before proceeding to more challenging exercises
Pulse rate (beats per minute) **Normal: 60–100 bpm** **Light activity: <110 bpm** **Intense activity: >110 bpm**	Notice your pulse rate or the number of beats per minute (bpm) by performing a simple stretching exercise. If it increases too much, it is an indication that you should start with simpler exercises that help you build enough stamina to exercise regularly. Consider exercises such as seated walking, seated swimming, or cat-cow stretch and pranayama for stamina-building and managing heart rate. Avoid high-impact activities like sun salutation, planks, or strength training in the beginning. Incorporate these kinds of exercises gradually into your workout routine to avoid unnecessary strain on your body.

Factors to determine your fitness level	How the factors help you determine your fitness needs and goals
	For seniors, a normal resting pulse ranges between 60 and 100 bpm (*Active and Resting Heart Rates*, n.d.). The normal range can vary based on factors such as overall health, fitness level, and any medications you might be taking. Your pulse rate can increase while doing daily chores or exercises. It's essential to monitor your pulse rate regularly, especially during rest and after physical activity, to ensure it remains within a healthy range. Any sustained elevation or irregularities in heart rate should prompt further evaluation by a healthcare professional to identify and address any underlying issues.
The circumference of your waist (measured at the level of your belly button) and the circumference of your hips	To determine your waist-to-hip ratio (WHR), divide the circumference of your waist by that of your hips. In general, a WHR above 0.80 for women and 0.94 for men indicates an increased risk of heart problems and diabetes (*Waist-Hip Ratio*, n.d.). Combining cardio exercises, Pilates, and strength training with a balanced diet and overall healthy lifestyle can help reduce WHR.
The number of wall push-ups you can do in a minute	The number of wall push-ups you can do in a minute can serve as a measure of upper body strength and muscular endurance. It indicates how many repetitions of the exercise you can perform within a specific time frame, reflecting your muscular stamina and ability to sustain effort over time. A higher number of wall push-ups suggests greater upper body strength, while a lower number may indicate that you

Factors to determine your fitness level	How the factors help you determine your fitness needs and goals
	need to focus on building strength with basic variations and progress gradually. It can help identify which muscle groups need more focus in your exercise routine. Seeing improvements over time indicates that your exercise regimen is effective in building strength and endurance.
Body mass index (BMI)	Your BMI can provide a rough estimate of whether you may have excess abdominal fat. A BMI of 25–29 indicates you are overweight, and a BMI of 30 or more means you are obese. If you have a higher BMI, including exercises to burn excess calories should be one of your primary fitness goals. Spinal twists, seated marching, seated cycling, and seated squats are some exercises you can do to decrease your BMI by promoting calorie burning, muscle building, and cardiovascular health.

Set SMART Goals

Prioritize your health goals based on whether you need to focus on weight management, muscle strengthening, flexibility and mobility enhancement, core strength and balance improvement, or stress and anxiety reduction. Consider what will best support your overall well-being and quality of life and plan SMART fitness goals for exercising (*How SMART Fitness Goals*, 2022):

- **Specific:** Clearly define what you want to accomplish with precise details and parameters. For example, "I will increase my upper body strength by performing 3 sets of 10 push-ups 3 times a week." This goal specifies the type of exercise (push-ups), sets a target number (3 sets of 10), and identifies frequency (3 times a week).

- **Measurable:** Set goals that can be tangibly measured to ensure clarity in your fitness journey. For example, "I will reduce my weight by 10 lbs. within 3 months." This goal quantifies progress by setting a measurable target (number of pounds lost) and specifies a tool for measurement (scale and body weight).

- **Attainable:** Set realistic and feasible goals that can be accomplished given your available resources and capabilities. For instance, "I will gradually work my way up to start walking with support by following a structured exercise plan over the next 3 months." This goal is realistic and achievable because it acknowledges the need for gradual progress and sets a reasonable timeline to get there.

- **Relevant:** Ensure that the goal aligns with your overall objectives and is meaningful and significant to you. For instance, "I will improve my cardiovascular health by doing 30 minutes of seated cycling and marching daily." This goal is relevant to the individual's overall health objective, focusing on cardiovascular fitness, which is important for overall well-being.

- **Time-bound:** Decide on a time frame for attaining your objectives. For instance, "I will increase my flexibility by performing yoga stretches daily with the goal of touching my toes comfortably in 3 months." This goal has a specific time frame (3 months) within which the individual is working to achieve increased flexibility, providing a sense of urgency and accountability.

Customized Workout Plan

Create a workout plan that suits your body and helps you progress at a comfortable pace. The maximum duration of your exercise session can vary between 20 and 30 minutes based on your stamina. In this section, we'll look at some points you should remember while creating a customized workout plan for yourself.

Be Mindful of the Duration and Frequency

Older adults aged 65 and above need at least 30 minutes of moderate-intensity workouts every day. Health and fitness experts also suggest seniors perform muscle-strengthening exercises at least 2 days a week and activities that improve balance and stability at least once a week. However, if you suffer from any health conditions, modify your exercise routine as advised by your healthcare provider (*How Much Physical Activity*, n.d.).

Start your exercise routine with a 5–10-minute warm-up of simple yoga stretches, meditation, or pranayama. End your session with restorative yoga.

Identify Preferences and Incorporate Fun Activities

Identify your favorite exercises to include in your chair fitness program. This can motivate you to exercise regularly.

To spice up your exercise session, play music and beautify your exercise space by adding some plants and letting in some sunshine and fresh air. Incorporate enjoyable activities such as listening to music or podcasts to make your workout routine more interesting and enjoyable.

Choose workouts and routines that target certain areas based on your health needs, such as strength, flexibility, balance, or cardiovascular health.

Experiment With Different Routines

Decide on the exercises you're going to incorporate according to your fitness needs and priorities. Keep adding and shuffling the exercises over time to ensure you derive maximum benefits. Integrate different exercise routines for a well-rounded approach to your fitness journey (Mayo Clinic Staff, 2023).

Modify Your Workouts and Be Responsive

Be sure to incorporate changes and variations to your exercise routine to meet your abilities and limits while ensuring safety and effectiveness. Use props, decrease holding time, or reduce the number of repetitions of a specific exercise to ensure you are responsive to your body and are not stressing it while exercising.

Track Your Progress

Tracking your progress regularly ensures that you are putting your efforts in the right direction and also gives you an idea of when to incorporate more challenging exercises. You can track your progress by noticing improvement in your flexibility, mobility, strength, and balance. You can also measure your waist and hip circumference, BMI, and pulse rate after an exercise, count the push-ups you can perform in a minute, and so on. You can keep an exercise journal to record and track your progress so you can stay motivated and focused on your fitness goals (Mayo Clinic Staff, 2023).

Seek Professional Advice

Though different exercise methods and programs are intended to help improve physical fitness, not all types of exercise are appropriate for all people. Consult with a fitness expert or healthcare practitioner for personalized advice, guidance, and support as you embark on your fitness journey.

Sample Exercise Routines

Some sample exercise plans are given below. Sample 1 is based on yoga, Sample 2 includes Pilates exercises, Sample 3 includes strength training, Sample 4 has cardio, and Sample 5 has integrated exercises. Before you start exercising, make sure to consult your doctor, identify your priorities, and set your fitness goals. You may have different fitness objectives every day, or they may change weekly. Measure your BMI and look closer at your muscle and joint flexibility. Do you need to manage weight, improve mobility, or both? Answering these questions will help you attain clarity in your goals.

Sample 1: Chair Yoga—5 days a week for 30 minutes

Day	Objective	Warm-up	Target exercise	Cool down
Monday	Flexibility	Shoulder rolls Arm, finger, and toe stretches	Seated side stretches Seated leg extensions	Butterfly pose
Tuesday	Core strength	Bee breath	Supine boat pose	Seated mountain pose
Wednesday	Spinal health	Seated cat-cow stretch	Prone boat pose	Diaphragmatic breathing
Thursday	Balance	Body scan meditation	Chair squats	Cooling breath Seated tree pose
Friday	Relaxation	Alternate nostril breathing	Legs up the wall pose	Loving-kindness meditation

Sample 2: Chair Pilates—5 days a week for 30 minutes

Day	Objective	Warm-up	Target exercise	Cool down
Monday	Core strength	Seated cat-cow stretch	Chair planks	Saw exercise on the bed
Tuesday	Flexibility	Seated spinal twist	Full body stretch	Seated forward fold
Wednesday	Balance and stability	Leg swings	Single leg circles	Roll-ups on the bed
Thursday	Posture	Shoulder rolls	The hundred	Side leg kicks on the bed
Friday	Injury prevention	Seated hip circles	Pelvic tilt	Full body stretch

Sample 3: Strength Training—2 days a week for 15–20 minutes

Day	Objective	Warm-up	Target exercise	Cool down
Tuesday	Arm muscle strengthening	Arm stretches Grip exercise	Bicep and tricep curls	Seated rows with a resistance band
Thursday	Leg muscle strengthening	Chair lunges	Chair squats	Seated chest presses

Sample 4: Chair Cardio—5 days a week for 30 minutes

Day	Objective	Warm-up	Target exercise	Cool down
Monday	Cardiovascular health	Seated marching	Seated high knee raises	Seated swimming
Tuesday	Improved respiratory function	Side leg tap	Seated bicycle crunches	Side arm cardio
Wednesday	Weight management	Seated cycling	Upper and lower tummy exercises Hip and thigh muscle toning exercise	Side leg tap
Thursday	Increased stamina	Seated bicycle crunches	Seated swimming	Side arm cardio
Friday	Better mental health	Jumping jacks with support	Dancing	Deep breathing

Sample 5: Integrated Chair Exercises—5 days a week for 20–30 minutes

Day	Objective	Exercise discipline	Warm-up	Target exercise	Cool down
Mon	Energy and vitality	Hatha yoga + restorative yoga	Alternate nostril breathing Om chanting/ prayer meditation	Seated sun salutation	Corpse pose Child's pose
Tue	Core strengthening	Yoga + Pilates	Shoulder rolls Cat-cow stretch	Standing tree pose with support	Child's pose
Wed	Heart health	Yoga + cardio	Pranayama Cooling breath	Bridge pose	Legs up the wall pose
Thu	Muscle building	Yoga + strength training	Seated side stretch Spinal twist on the chair	Boat pose Chair squats	Bee breath
Fri	Joint health	Yoga + strength training	Ankle rotation Wrist rotation	Seated Pilates teaser	Ankle rotations Leg swings

Day	Objective	Exercise discipline	Warm-up	Target exercise	Cool down
			Leg swings		Diaphragmatic breathing

As you plan your exercise schedule, remember to start simple, consider your level of mobility, and work out for manageable lengths of time. Do not ignore the fact that a healthy meal provides you the energy you need to get a good workout. A healthy diet and regular exercise complement one another.

Healthy Eating to Complement Your Fitness Routine

Eat a low-calorie diet filled with protein, minerals, and antioxidant-rich foods. Your bone density and muscle mass reduce with age, so getting the right amounts of calcium and vitamin D is important for bone health. Dairy products, leafy greens, and tofu are good sources of calcium. Vitamin D, which helps the body absorb calcium, can be obtained through sunlight exposure as well as from sources like fatty fish, fortified dairy products, and supplements.

You can ensure you're getting essential nutrients by eating fruits, vegetables, whole grains, and lean proteins. Vegetables and fruits are good sources of antioxidants, the compounds that protect the body from diseases like arthritis, heart ailments, and cancer. Including antioxidant-rich foods in your diet, such as berries, nuts, and leafy greens, can help combat oxidative stress and promote long-term health and well-being. Antioxidants are vital for reducing the risk of chronic diseases and promoting overall health.

Legumes like lentils, beans, and peas are rich in fiber, protein, and minerals. Avoiding excessive alcohol consumption and not smoking are also important for maintaining bone density and overall health. Eating foods high in protein, fiber, minerals, and antioxidants helps with healthy weight management (Beyer, 2019).

Monounsaturated and polyunsaturated fats like omega-3 and omega-6 fatty acids, which can be found in foods like fatty fish, avocados, nuts, and seeds, are important for your functional fitness. On the other hand, you want to try and avoid foods that contain trans fats and saturated fats because they increase the risk of heart disease.

This chapter offered personalized chair fitness routines designed to enhance muscle tone, increase range of motion, and boost cardiovascular fitness all while prioritizing safety and accessibility. From shoulder rolls and spinal twists to chair marches and bicep curls, these exercises have been incorporated to offer you a diverse tool kit for building strength and resilience in the comfort of your chair.

Be consistent and patient to achieve maximum positive outcomes of chair exercises. Start slowly, listen to your body, and gradually progress as your strength and confidence grow. Always consult a healthcare professional before beginning any new exercise program, especially if you have underlying health concerns or mobility limitations. Be creative, have clear fitness goals, and take proactive steps toward maintaining independence, promoting vitality, and enjoying an active lifestyle well into your golden years. Next in the bonus chapter included in this book, you'll find a fun and invigorating 28-day yoga challenge to put all your newfound fitness knowledge into action.

Bonus Chapter:

28-Day Yoga Challenge for Flexibility, Mental Clarity, and Overall Health

Once you have started exercising regularly, it is time to challenge yourself a bit more. Setting new goals frequently throughout your exercise journey ensures your fitness level is continuously progressing. Here is a 28-day yoga challenge to help you attain flexibility, enjoy mental calmness and relaxation, and improve your health and vitality. You may start noticing the changes within the first 5 days, but push yourself and continue the challenge for all 28 days!

Be responsive to your body's signals, use yoga props, relax, and don't forget to eat right and sleep tight.

Day	Fitness goal	Warm-up	Target exercise	Cool down
1	Mental and physical relaxation	Prayer meditation	Corpse pose	Mantra meditation
2	Full body stretch	Neck rotations	Seated sun salutation	Seated mountain pose
3	Hand Exercises	Finger rotations Wrist circles	Chair planks	Arm stretches

Day	Fitness goal	Warm-up	Target exercise	Cool down
4	Back exercises	Cat-cow stretch on chair	Bridge pose Cobra pose	Butterfly pose
5	Engaging the shoulders	Shoulder rolls	Warrior II	Downward-facing dog

Did you feel a positive change in your overall health and flexibility? Now get ready for another 23 days...

Day	Fitness goal	Warm-up	Target exercise	Cool down
6	Mental clarity	Prayer mediation Victorious breath	Loving-kindness meditation	Child's pose
7	Back exercises	Cat-cow stretch	Bridge pose on bed Cobra pose on bed	Butterfly pose on bed
8	Knee exercises	Seated knee lifts	Warrior II	Reclining hand-to-big-toe
9	Morning affirmation	Prayer meditation	Affirmation meditation	Arm stretches Leg extensions Forward folds

Day	Fitness goal	Warm-up	Target exercise	Cool down
10	Yoga for tight hips	Easy pose with prana mudra	Bridge pose on the bed	Seated pigeon pose
11	Yoga for vitality	Cooling breath	Sun Salutation	Boat pose on the bed
12	Yoga for self-care	Loving-kindness meditation Seated mountain pose	Face yoga	Body scan meditation
13	Bedtime yoga	Sukhasana with dhyana mudra	Legs up the wall pose	Corpse pose
14	Yoga for core strength	The hundred	Chair planks	Tree pose with support
15	Yoga for preventing and managing sciatica pain	Cat-cow stretch	Downward-facing dog	Seated pigeon pose
16	Spinal flexibility	Seated spinal twists	Cobra pose on the bed	Full body stretch
17	Heart health	Diaphragmatic breathing	Jumping jacks with support	Fish pose
18	Healthy gut	Apana mudra	Boat pose on bed	Seated forward folds

Day	Fitness goal	Warm-up	Target exercise	Cool down
			Prone bow pose on bed	
19	Managing arthritis pain	Wrist circles Ankle rotations	Warrior II on a chair Knee presses on the bed	Leg swings
20	Mental calmness	Affirmation meditation	Seated forward folds	Body scan meditation
21	Balance and stability	Chair pose	Squats with support	Seated calf raises
22	Mental and physical relaxation	Prayer meditation	Corpse pose on bed	Mantra meditation
23	Healthy gut	Seated forward folds	Boat pose on bed Prone bow pose on bed	Apana mudra
24	Yoga for tight hips	Seated pigeon pose on a chair	Bridge pose on the bed	Padmasana with prana mudra
25	Managing arthritis pain	Wrist circles Ankle rotations	Warrior II on a chair	Leg swings

Day	Fitness goal	Warm-up	Target exercise	Cool down
			Knee presses on the bed	
26	Heart health	Diaphragmatic breathing	Jumping jacks with support	Fish pose
27	Balance and stability	Chair pose	Squats with support	Seated calf raises
28	Spinal flexibility	Seated spinal twists	Cobra pose on the bed	Full body stretch

Enjoy this journey of self-discovery and well-being through daily yoga practice by focusing on strength, flexibility, and inner peace for 28 days. Let each session enrich your body, mind, and soul and set you on the path to a sustainable yoga journey. Be kind to yourself, listen to your body's signals, and take breaks if you feel any discomfort.

Conclusion

Chair Yoga and Beyond is a comprehensive and accessible guide to maintaining fitness and mobility from the comfort of a chair. With its clear instructions and science-based exercises, readers can easily incorporate these movements into their daily workout routines. By emphasizing the importance of movement regardless of physical limitations, this book has empowered you to take charge of your health and well-being. Whether for seniors, those with mobility challenges, or anyone seeking convenient, low-impact exercise options, this resource offers a pathway to improved strength, flexibility, and posture, enhanced cardiovascular health, and overall vitality.

Embracing the Benefits of Chair-Based Fitness

A chair-based fitness program is a gentle yet effective springboard for increased mobility, strength, and overall well-being for seniors, individuals with limited mobility, or people facing chronic illnesses. Incorporating a chair into your workouts opens the door to movements you may not otherwise be able to perform. This inclusive approach promotes confidence and independence while facilitating a sense of accomplishment and improved quality of life.

Exercising stimulates your nervous system to release happy hormones like endorphins and dopamine and inhibits the production of stress hormones. So even when life seems difficult, smile and exercise your way to a happy, stress-free life.

Take Care of Your Safety and Well-Being

Be attuned to your body's signals and do not overexert yourself to get fast results. Put in your honest efforts and be kind to your muscles, bones, and joints with careful movements and plenty of time to rest and recover between workouts.

Integrate Yoga, Pilates, Cardio, and Strength Training for Holistic Health Benefits

The use of a chair and bed in yoga has made it more inclusive of people with different fitness levels. Using yoga props such as cushions, bolsters, straps, and blocks can enhance your practice, extending its scope and depth by providing support and stability and making challenging poses more accessible.

While yoga alone provides many physical, mental, and spiritual benefits, integrating other forms of exercise can further enrich your health and fitness. Apart from enhancing muscle and joint flexibility and strength, yoga emphasizes the connection between the mind and body through breath awareness and mindful movement. This holistic approach can help reduce stress, improve mental clarity, and enhance overall well-being.

Pilates, a discipline that is inspired by yoga and martial arts, is useful in developing core strength and flexibility. Pilates focuses on controlled movements, proper alignment, and breathing techniques to improve overall strength, coordination, and balance. The practice engages the core muscles and the spine and enhances your posture.

Resistance training improves muscular health and helps prevent injuries due to bone and muscle loss in seniors caused by osteoporosis and can help reverse the effects of aging. Using 3–5 lb. dumbbells for bicep and tricep curls is safe for seniors. Using excessively heavy weights (more than 5 lbs.) is not advisable as they could lead to sprains or other injuries.

Cardio exercises make your heart beat faster, which leads to improved circulation and a faster supply of oxygen and nutrients to your muscles and organs while also removing waste products. As a result, your heart becomes stronger and more efficient over time, reducing the overall stress on the heart during physical activity and at rest.

Exercising your joints leads to independence and overall health. A sedentary lifestyle can lead to friction and joint inflammation. This may aggravate health problems and cause redness, swelling, and arthritis. Exercise is important to reverse the effects of reduced blood flow and less lubrication in joints with age.

Eat a Balanced Diet to Stay Healthy and Support Your Exercise Regimen

Apart from exercising, there are other measures you can take to support joint health. A balanced diet goes hand in hand with exercising. A diet rich in lean proteins, whole grains, fruits, and vegetables provides essential nutrients for overall health, including bone and muscle strength. Eating a low-fat, high-fiber, high-protein diet supports healthy weight management and keeps you active. However, if you are living with a health condition, you need to follow the recommendations of your healthcare provider.

In addition to eating a healthy, balanced diet, it's also important to stay hydrated. When combined with regular exercise, hydration and nutrition contribute to improved physical performance, enhanced recovery, and better management of chronic conditions. Maintaining a balanced diet and proper hydration can aid in weight management, promote cognitive function, and reduce the risk of chronic diseases such as diabetes and heart disease. Together, these lifestyle habits support a healthier, more vibrant life.

Breathe Deeply and Meditate to Foster Calmness, Reduce Stress, and Enhance Mental Clarity

Deep breathing regulates the nervous system, encourages relaxation and mindfulness, alleviates stress, and helps maintain good sleep hygiene. Practicing mindful movement during seated workouts and concentrating on the sensations of movement and breath deepens relaxation and awareness, brings harmony, and provides holistic health benefits. Keep a calm mind through pranayama and meditation techniques mentioned in this book.

A good sleep schedule is important for your overall health and vitality. Consistent sleep schedules and bedtime routines such as reading, listening to music, or praying before bedtime promote quality sleep. Quality sleep provides energy, relieves stress in muscles and joints, and can be instrumental in exercising regularly.

Plan Your Exercise Regimen Carefully and Mindfully

A result-oriented approach to exercising is well-planned and integrates the most effective aspects of various exercise disciplines. Remember to assess your fitness level by checking your mobility status, strength, pulse rate, body weight, waist-hip ratio, and BMI frequently and before planning your schedule. Challenging yourself when you have shown progress in a certain area is crucial for motivation and continued improvement. Start your exercise session with 5–10 minutes of warming up and end it with a cool-down session of the same duration. Perform the more intense exercises in between the warm-up and cool down and incorporate gentle deep breathing into all exercises. Do restorative poses, take breaks, and use yoga props for comfort.

Incorporating a range of activities while being consistent can help you avoid boredom and plateauing. Identify your favorite exercises, hobbies, or fitness methods to include in your chair fitness program to make it more interesting. Try different combinations of exercises, routines, and formats to see what works best for you. Incorporating things you enjoy such as music, podcasts, or audiobooks can help you look forward to your workout sessions and get more out of them.

Do not ignore your body's signals like pain or discomfort and do not hesitate to change your fitness routine as necessary to avoid burnout, injury, or overtraining.

Essential Exercises to Keep in Mind

This table is adapted from Banerjee, 2022:

Health issue/fitness goal	Exercise
Shoulder problems	Shoulder rolls, spinal twist, mountain pose
Neck pain	Neck rotations, gentle neck stretches
Back pain	Bridge pose, cat-cow stretch, butterfly pose
Knee pain	Butterfly pose, triangle pose, gentle knee presses
Heart health	Cardio exercises like seated walking, seated swimming, etc. Pranayama, meditation
Mental relaxation	Pranayama, meditation
Muscular relaxation	Corpse pose, legs up the wall pose, child's pose

Enjoy the newfound strength, flexibility, and mindfulness obtained from your chair-based fitness adventure as it enables you to live a full and active life in your golden years. I hope you adopt chair-based activities as a long-term method to increase your agility, mobility, strength, and general quality of life and instill a sense of independence and empowerment. Happy exercising!

References

Active and resting heart rates: How to know what your numbers should be as a senior. (n.d.). *Senior Helpers.* https://www.seniorhelpers.com/ca/concord/resources/blogs/understanding-active-and-resting-heart-rates-in-seniors/#:~:text=A%20healthy%20resting%20heart%20rate

American Council on Exercise. (2013, October 11). Core anatomy: Muscles of the core. *Ace.* https://www.acefitness.org/fitness-certifications/ace-answers/exam-preparation-blog/3562/core-anatomy-muscles-of-the-core/

Arhanta Yoga. (2020, March 26). *Daily pranayama practice | Arhanta Yoga* [Video]. YouTube. https://www.youtube.com/watch?v=-r9HOpSkI1E&t=739s

Banerjee, T. (2022, June 21). Yes, yoga can alleviate joint pain. Gentle asanas that will ensure a comfortable life. *The Economic Times | Panache.* https://economictimes.indiatimes.com/magazines/panache/yes-yoga-can-alleviate-joint-pain-gentle-asanas-that-will-ensure-a-comfortable-life/articleshow/92208248.cms

Beyer, M. (2019, February 24). *What diet is best for older adults?* Medical News Today. https://www.medicalnewstoday.com/articles/324514

Boccia, M., Piccardi, L., & Guariglia, P. (2015). The meditative mind: A comprehensive meta-analysis of MRI studies. *BioMed research international, 2015,* 1–11. https://doi.org/10.1155/2015/419808

Bramble, L.-A. (2021, April 19). *Static vs. dynamic stretching: What are they and which should you do?* Hospital for Special Surgery. https://www.hss.edu/article_static_dynamic_stretching.asp#:~:text=Static%20stretches%20are%20those%20in

Brand, M. (2019, October 9). 15 quotes of active adults over 50. *Brand Fitness*. https://www.brandfitness.ca/blog/15-quotes-of-active-adults-over-50

Calculate your body mass index. (n.d.). National Heart, Lung, and Blood Institute. https://www.nhlbi.nih.gov/health/educational/lose_wt/BMI/bmicalc.htm

Chair yoga and why seated yoga poses are good for you. (2023, January 1). Lifespan. https://www.lifespan.org/lifespan-living/chair-yoga-and-why-seated-yoga-poses-are-good-you

Christian. (2023, December 12). *5 easy seated abdominal exercises to strengthen your core.* Kustom Strength. https://kustomkitgymequipment.com/blogs/news/seated-abdominal-exercises/

Cronkleton, E. (2021, February 11). *Face yoga for inner and outer radiance?* Healthline. https://www.healthline.com/health/fitness-exercise/face-yoga#takeaway

Denish Obeiro, A. (n.d.). *Aloo Denish Obiero quotes.* Goodreads. https://www.goodreads.com/quotes/11966448-rigidity-invites-vulnerability-flexibility-breeds-adaptability#:~:text=Rigidity%20invites%20vulnerability%3B%20flexibility%20breeds%20adaptability

8 best core exercises for seniors. (n.d.). Lifeline. https://www.lifeline.ca/en/resources/core-exercises-for-seniors/

8 great exercises to safeguard your spine. (n.d.). *Spine Group Beverly Hills.* https://www.spinegroupbeverlyhills.com/blog/8-great-exercises-to-safeguard-your-spine#:~:text=Stretching%20and%20exercising%20your%20backSS

Ennis, K. (2023, November 14). *5 best balance exercises for seniors: Building strength and stability* [Video]. YouTube. https://www.youtube.com/watch?v=swq5if3c-gg

Exercise and the heart. (n.d.). Johns Hopkins Medicine. https://www.hopkinsmedicine.org/health/wellness-and-prevention/exercise-and-the-heart#:~:text=Improves%20the%20muscles

FitnessBlender. (2012, October 12). *Pilates infused cool down and stretch workout to tone and lengthen* [Video]. YouTube. https://www.youtube.com/watch?v=NuagzNoRXII

Futurefit. (n.d.). Use imagery to help with posture. *Future Fit.* https://www.futurefit.co.uk/blog/use-imagery-to-help-with-posture/#:~:text=The%20following%20are%20examples%20of

Galantino, M. L., Green, L., DeCesari, J. A., MacKain, N. A., Rinaldi, S. M., Stevens, M. E., Wurst, V. R., Marsico, R., Nell, M., & Mao, J. J. (2012). Safety and feasibility of modified chair-yoga on functional outcome among elderly at risk for falls. *International journal of yoga, 5*(2), 146–150. https://journals.lww.com/ijoy/fulltext/2012/05020/safety_and_feasibility_of_modified_chair_yoga_on.12.aspx

Helmer, J. (n.d.). *Chair yoga poses.* WebMD. https://www.webmd.com/fitness-exercise/features/chair-yoga-poses

Horne, B. (2023, September 7). *Chair yoga for seniors: Poses and how to try.* Medical News Today. https://www.medicalnewstoday.com/articles/chair-yoga-for-seniors#does-it-work

How much physical activity do older adults need? (n.d.). Centers for Disease Control and Prevention. https://www.cdc.gov/physicalactivity/basics/older_adults/index.htm#:~:text=Adults%20aged%2065%20and%20older

How SMART fitness goals can help you get healthier. (2022, November 16). Cleveland Clinic Health Essentials. https://health.clevelandclinic.org/smart-fitness-goals

ildan, M. M. (n.d.). *Mehmet Murat ildan quotes.* Goodreads. https://www.goodreads.com/quotes/8980760-life-continuously-shoots-arrows-at-you-to-survive-be-flexible

Jain, R. (2023, October 8). *Complete guide to mudras: Benefits and use in yoga, meditation & chakra balancing.* Arhanta Yoga. https://www.arhantayoga.org/blog/complete-guide-to-mudras-and-benefits/

Jefferson, T. (n.d.). *Thomas Jefferson quotes.* Goodreads. https://www.goodreads.com/quotes/1361034-if-you-want-something-you-ve-never-had-you-must-be

Joanna Soh Official. (2017, February 9). *5-minute inner thighs & abs in bed | Joanna Soh* [Video]. YouTube. https://www.youtube.com/watch?v=bxR1VnIffCU

Joints. (n.d.). Cleveland Clinic. https://my.clevelandclinic.org/health/body/25137-joints

Kabat-Zinn, J. (n.d.). *Jon Kabat-Zinn quotes.* QuoteFancy. https://quotefancy.com/quote/1283051/Jon-Kabat-Zinn-Mindfulness-means-being-awake-It-means-knowing-what-you-are-doing

Kabat-Zinn, J. (2023, February 10). *This loving-kindness meditation is a radical act of love.* Mindful. https://www.mindful.org/this-loving-kindness-meditation-is-a-radical-act-of-love/

Kain, C. (n.d.). *The surprising benefits of chair yoga.* Kripalu Center for Yoga & Health. https://kripalu.org/resources/surprising-benefits-chair-yoga

Kingsford, J. (n.d.). *Jana Kingsford quotes.* Goodreads. https://www.goodreads.com/quotes/7966823-balance-is-not-something-you-find-it-s-something-you-create

Kloubec, J. (2011). Pilates: How does it work and who needs it? *Muscles, ligaments and tendons journal, 1*(2), 61–66. https://www.ncbi.nlm.nih.gov/pmc/articles/PMC3666467/#: ~:text=Pilates%20uses%20a%20combination%20of

LaLanne, J. (n.d.). *Jack LaLanne quotes.* AZ Quotes. https://www.azquotes.com/quote/797854

M, A. (2021, December 17). Creating an exercise plan for seniors - 6 tips. *FitSW.* https://www.fitsw.com/blog/creating-an-exercise-plan-for-seniors-6-tips/

The Man Flow Yoga Team. (n.d.). How to use cardio and yoga to take your fitness to the next level. *Man Flow Yoga.* https://manflowyoga.com/blog/how-to-use-cardio-and-yoga-to-take-your-fitness-to-the-next-level/#:~:text=If%20losing%20weight%20is%20your

Manheim, A. (2023, September 28). How to breathe the Pilates way. *Pilates Anytime.* https://www.pilatesanytime.com/blog/more/how-to-breathe-the-pilates-way#:~:text=On%20an%20inhale%2C%20breathe%20into

Mayo Clinic Staff. (2023, December 5). *Fitness program: 5 steps to get started.* Mayo Clinic. https://www.mayoclinic.org/healthy-lifestyle/fitness/in-depth/fitness/art-20048269

Mayo Clinic Staff. (2024, January 31). *Sciatica.* Mayo Clinic. https://www.mayoclinic.org/diseases-conditions/sciatica/symptoms-causes/syc-20377435#:~:text=Sciatica%20refers%20to%20pain%20that

McGee, K. (2022, November 21). *11 types of yoga: A breakdown of the major styles.* Mindbodygreen. https://www.mindbodygreen.com/articles/the-11-major-types-of-yoga-explained-simply

McGonigle, A. (2022, September 26). *5 ways to practice crow pose.* Yoga Journal. https://www.yogajournal.com/practice/5-ways-to-practice-crow-pose/

MasterClass. (2021, June 7). *The meaning of Om: How to use Om in your yoga practice.* https://www.masterclass.com/articles/what-does-om-mean-explained

Meditation. (n.d.). Cleveland Clinic. https://my.clevelandclinic.org/health/articles/17906-meditation

Mindfulness. (n.d.). Psychology Today. https://www.psychologytoday.com/intl/basics/mindfulness

Moonaz, S., Bartlett, S. J., & Bingham III, C. O. (2019, January 8). *Yoga for arthritis.* Johns Hopkins Arthritis Center. https://www.hopkinsarthritis.org/patient-corner/disease-management/yoga-for-arthritis/

Parkerton, M. (2023, August 17). Treat your heart right: 125 sayings and quotes about heart disease. *Parade.* https://parade.com/1187612/michelle-parkerton/quotes-about-heart-disease/

A patient's guide to anatomy and function of the spine. (n.d.). University of Maryland Medical Center. https://www.umms.org/ummc/health-services/orthopedics/services/spine/patient-guides/anatomy-function

Pilates and posture: Strengthening your core for optimal alignment and balance. (2023, July 22). *Pilates Reformers Plus.* https://pilatesreformersplus.com/blogs/news/pilates-and-posture-strengthening-your-core-for-optimal-alignment-and-balance

Pilates, J. (n.d.). *Joseph Pilates quotes*. QuoteFancy. https://quotefancy.com/quote/1559817/Joseph-Pilates-I-must-be-right-Never-an-aspirin-Never-injured-a-day-in-my-life-The-whole

Pilatesology. (2012, January 13). *Pilates teaser exercise with Alisa Wyatt* [Video]. YouTube. https://www.youtube.com/watch?v=ptGlPgInTrY

Pizer, A. (2018, January 18). Yoga for strength: 9 of yoga's best strength-building poses. *Liforme*. https://liforme.com/blogs/blog/yoga-for-strength

Raypole, C. (2022, December 5). *How to do a body scan meditation (and why you should)*. Healthline. https://www.healthline.com/health/body-scan-meditation#:~:text=The%20body%20scan%20is%20a

Royal Free London NHS Foundation Trust. (2017, June 30). *Seated pelvic tilt* [Video]. YouTube. https://www.youtube.com/watch?v=SlzYz7SQns4

SarahBethYoga. (2022, September 19). *At home cardio + yoga | Let's talk about it* [Video]. YouTube. https://www.youtube.com/watch?v=Z2N3UKozKOY

Scotti, A., & Ritchey, C. (2023, July 26). 35 fitness quotes to push you through your toughest workouts. *Men's Health*. https://www.menshealth.com/fitness/a19547200/best-fitness-quotes-of-all-time/

Seguin, R., & Nelson, M. E. (2003). The benefits of strength training for older adults. *American journal of preventive medicine*, *25*(3), 141–149. https://doi.org/10.1016/s0749-3797(03)00177-6

SeniorShape Fitness. (2021, September 13). *Chair Pilates for seniors & beginners || Gentle Pilates workout with stretching* [Video]. YouTube. https://www.youtube.com/watch?v=jsFzFiyDqBs

SeniorShape Fitness. (2023, February 6). *Chair exercises for seniors // 10 minute cardio workout* [Video]. YouTube. https://www.youtube.com/watch?v=f-V31VugkHw

SilverSneakers. (2021, April 8). *5 seated Pilates exercise movements for seniors | SilverSneakers* [Video]. YouTube. https://www.youtube.com/watch?v=U73T-XiIm9Y

Six tips for safe stretches. (2019, December 11). Harvard Health Publishing. https://www.health.harvard.edu/staying-healthy/six-tips-for-safe-stretches

Tannous, O. (2021, June 30). 10 tips for a healthier spine. *MedStar Health*. https://www.medstarhealth.org/blog/tips-for-healthy-spine

Tiernan, C., Lysack, C., Neufeld, S., & Lichtenberg, P. A. (2013). Community engagement: An essential component of well-being in older African-American adults. *The international journal of aging & human development,* *77*(3), 233–257. https://journals.sagepub.com/doi/10.2190/AG.77.3.d

Vago, D. R., & Silbersweig, D. A. (2012). Self-awareness, self-regulation, and self-transcendence (S-ART): a framework for understanding the neurobiological mechanisms of mindfulness. *Frontiers in human neuroscience,* *6.* https://www.frontiersin.org/articles/10.3389/fnhum.2012.00296/full

Vo, K. (2024, March 29). *100 mindfulness quotes to go from stress to blessed at work.* FlexOS. https://www.flexos.work/tools/mindfulness-quotes-for-work

Waist-hip ratio (WHR) and waist circumference. (n.d.). Maastricht UMC+ Nutritional Assessment. https://nutritionalassessment.mumc.nl/en/waist-hip-ratio-whr-and-waist-circumference#:~:text=The%20Waist%2Dto%2Dhip%20Ratio

Why it's good to accompany yoga with strength training. (n.d.). McClure Fitness. https://mcclurefitness.com/why-its-good-to-accompany-yoga-with-strength-training/

Yao, C.-T., Lee, B.-O., Hong, H., & Su, Y.-C. (2023). Effect of chair yoga therapy on functional fitness and daily life activities among older female adults with knee osteoarthritis in Taiwan: A quasi-experimental study. *Healthcare*, *11*(7), 1024. https://doi.org/10.3390/healthcare11071024

Yoga Vista (aka YogaJP). (2013, September 29). *Actively aging with energizing chair yoga - Seniors get moving with Sherry Zak Morris, C-IAYT* [Video]. YouTube. https://www.youtube.com/watch?v=k4ST1j9PfrA

Yoopod. (2015, August 11). *Swan dive Pilates exercise from yoopod.com* [Video]. YouTube. https://www.youtube.com/watch?v=EYmc4itM99Y

Image References

Aurelius, M. (2021, January 27). *Couple practicing yoga.* [Image]. Pexels. https://www.pexels.com/photo/couple-practicing-yoga-6787519/

Bolovtsova, K. (2020, April 26). *A woman doing a yoga exercise on a chair* [Image]. Pexels. https://www.pexels.com/photo/a-woman-doing-a-yoga-exercise-on-a-chair-7113446/

Engin_Akyurt. (2023, September 13). *Weight, dumbbell, strength image* [Image]. Pixabay. https://pixabay.com/photos/weight-dumbbell-strength-arm-force-8246973/

Geralt. (2024, March 11). *AI generated seniors walk* [Image]. Pixabay. https://pixabay.com/illustrations/ai-generated-seniors-walk-elderly-8627316/

Kampus Production. (2021a, January 13). *An elderly man working out* [Image]. Pexels. https://www.pexels.com/photo/an-elderly-man-working-out-6922152/

Kampus Production. (2021b, March 25). *A man in blue sweater wearing eyeglasses doing exercise* [Image]. Pexels. https://www.pexels.com/photo/a-man-in-blue-sweater-wearing-eyeglasses-doing-exercise-7551627/

Krukau, Y. (2020, November 4). *A therapist massaging the woman's back* [Image]. Pexels. https://www.pexels.com/photo/a-therapist-massaging-the-woman-s-back-5793804/

Krukau, Y. (2021, February 13). *Elderly people working out at the gym* [Image]. Pexels. https://www.pexels.com/photo/elderly-people-working-out-at-the-gym-6815699/

Nilov, M. (2021a, February 27). *An elderly woman doing a yoga* [Image]. Pexels. https://www.pexels.com/photo/an-elderly-woman-doing-a-yoga-6975760/

Nilov, M. (2021b, April 13). *Elderly woman doing yoga* [Image]. Pexels. https://www.pexels.com/photo/elderly-woman-doing-yoga-7500668/

Nilov, M. (2021c, April 16). *An elderly man doing exercise* [Image]. Pexels. https://www.pexels.com/photo/an-elderly-man-doing-exercise-7530370/

RDNE Stock project. (2021, July 11). *A man meditating in the garden* [Image]. Pexels. https://www.pexels.com/photo/a-man-meditating-in-the-garden-8710824/

Roma, A. (2021, April 12). *Woman exercising with elastic loop near crop partner* [Image]. Pexels. https://www.pexels.com/photo/woman-exercising-with-elastic-loop-near-crop-partner-7479778/

Samkov, I. (2021, January 30). *A woman doing nostril breathing* [Image]. Pexels. https://www.pexels.com/photo/a-woman-doing-nostril-breathing-6648567/

Shuraeva, A. (2020, October 26). *Photo of a woman with gray hair meditating* [Image]. Pexels. https://www.pexels.com/photo/photo-of-a-woman-with-gray-hair-meditating-5704848/

Shvets, A. (2020a, August 2). *Flexible slim woman doing bridge yoga asana on toes in sunny studio* [Image]. Pexels. https://www.pexels.com/photo/flexible-slim-woman-doing-bridge-yoga-asana-on-toes-in-sunny-studio-5012074/

Shvets, A. (2020b, August 9). *Sporty elderly man training with dumbbells* [Image]. Pexels. https://www.pexels.com/photo/sporty-elderly-man-training-with-dumbbells-5067739/

Thirdman. (2021, February 25). *Close-up shot of a person in a mudra pose* [Image]. Pexels. https://www.pexels.com/photo/close-up-shot-of-a-person-in-a-mudra-pose-6958260/

Wave, M. (2021, January 10). *Flexible woman doing Jathara Parivartanasana posture* [Image]. Pexels. https://www.pexels.com/photo/flexible-woman-doing-jathara-parivartanasana-posture-6454023/

Wellness Gallery Catalyst Foundation. (2022, May 9). *Group of elderly people exercising together* [Image]. Pexels. https://www.pexels.com/photo/group-of-elderly-people-exercising-together-12085616/